LESLEY L`

EAT RIGHT! BURN FAT!

Miracle Benefits of Apple Cider Vinegar

2017

Copyright 2017 by LESLEY LYNN HUDSON. All rights reserved.

All rights Reserved. No part of this publication or the information in it may be quoted from or reproduced in any form by means such as printing, scanning, photocopying or otherwise without prior written permission of the copyright holder.

Disclaimer and Terms of Use: Effort has been made to ensure that the information in this book is accurate and complete, however, the author and the publisher do not warrant the accuracy of the information, text, and graphics contained within the book due to the rapidly changing nature of science, research, known and unknown facts and the internet.

All information is intended only to help you cooperate with your doctor, in your efforts toward desirable weight levels and health. Only your doctor can determine what is right for you. In addition to regular checkups and medical supervision, from your doctor, before starting any other weight loss program, you should consult with your personal physician.

The Author and the publisher do not hold any responsibility for errors, omissions or contrary interpretation of the subject matter herein. This book is presented solely for motivational and informational purposes only.

Contents

Introduction 7

Chapter 1: What Is Apple Cider Vinegar? 10

Chapter 2: How to Make Apple Cider Vinegar 12

Chapter 3: Tips When Making and using Apple Cider Vinegar 14

Chapter 4: Apple Cider Vinegar Benefits 17

    HELPS TO REGULATE BLOOD SUGAR 18
    REDUCES CHOLESTEROL AND TRIGLYCERIDE LEVELS 18
    PROMOTES WEIGHT LOSS 19
    FIGHTS CANCER 19
    STIMULATES DIGESTION AND MINERAL ABSORPTION 19
    UTILIZATION OF IRON 20
    GREAT SOURCE OF POTASSIUM 20
    PROMOTES HEALTHY DETOXIFICATION 20

- *EASY TO USE* 20
- *SKIN CARE* 21
    TONE YOUR SKIN 21
    CLEANSE YOUR PORES 22
    EASE A SUNBURN 23
    MINIMIZE PSORIASIS 25
    REDUCE THE APPEARANCE OF FACIAL "MASKS." 26

- *HAIR CARE* 27
    HELP THINNING HAIR 29
    BEAT DANDRUFF 30
    MAKE YOUR HAIR RINSE 31
    MAKE YOUR SHAMPOO 32
    MAKE YOUR CONDITIONER 33
    COMBAT BALDNESS 33
    IMPROVE HAIR POROSITY 35
    DETANGLE HAIR 36
    REDUCE FRIZZ 37
    PREVENT SPLIT ENDS 38
    KILL AND PREVENT HEAD LICE 39

- PROMOTE HAIR GROWTH ... 40
- ADD SHINE ... 41
- PROMOTE SCALP HEALTH ... 42

➤ **STRESS & ODOR** ... 43
- MAKE YOUR DEODORANT ... 43

➤ **WONDERS WITH WEIGHT LOSS** ... 44
- APPLE CIDER VINEGAR KEEPS PEOPLE FEELING SATIATED ... 45
- APPLE CIDER VINEGAR HELPS IMPROVE PROTEIN UTILIZATION ... 45
- APPLE CIDER VINEGAR HELPS EFFECTIVELY BURN FATS IN THE STOMACH ... 46
- APPLE CIDER VINEGAR CAN IMPROVE UTILIZATION OF IRON ... 46
- APPLE CIDER VINEGAR INCREASES YOUR INTEREST TO WHOLE FOODS ... 46
- APPLE CIDER VINEGAR CONTAINS POTASSIUM ... 47

➤ **APPETITE AND FAT LOSS** ... 47

➤ **DETOXIFICATION** ... 49
- FEWER TOXINS, LESS WEIGHT ... 49

➤ **DETOXIFY YOUR LIVER** ... 49

➤ **CURES AND REMEDIES** ... 52
- ACHES, PAINS & BITES ... 52
- SOOTHE STOMACHACHES ... 53
- EASE A SORE THROAT ... 53
- SOOTHE SINUSITIS ... 54
- RELIEVE LEG CRAMPS ... 55
- RELIEVE MUSCLE STIFFNESS ... 57
- LESSEN JOINT PAIN ... 58
- ALLEVIATE HEADACHES ... 59
- REDUCE SWELLING ... 60
- RELIEVE EARACHES ... 61
- EASE BACKACHES ... 62
- RELIEVE BURNS ... 64
- HEAL BRUISES ... 65
- RELIEVE INSECT BITES ... 66

➤ **ACNE** ... 67

➤ **EASE INDIGESTION** ... 69

➤ **AVOID BACTERIAL CYSTITIS** ... 70

- SPEED UP METABOLISM 71
- ACID REFLUX 72
- REDUCE FLATULENCE 72

Chapter 5: Health Risks Associated with Apple Cider Vinegar Diet 74

Chapter 6: Cooking with Apple Cider 76

HEALTHY DRINKS 76
- 1. APPLE CIDER VINEGAR DRINK 76
- 2. ALMOND LATTE 78
- 3. GREEN TEA GINGER HOT TONIC 79
- 4. REFRESHING APPLE LEMON GINGER DRINK 80

APPLE CIDER VINEGAR DRESSING AND SAUCES 82
- 5. CLASSIC APPLE CIDER VINEGAR DRESSING 82
- 6. LOVELY APPLE SAUCE 84
- 7. EXQUISITE CREAMY POPPY SEED DRESSING 85

SALADS 86
- 8. APPETIZING POTATO SALAD WITH CORNICHONS AND RADISHES 86
- 9. DIETARY LETTUCE SALAD WITH APPLE DRESSING 88
- 10. FRESH COLLARD GREEN SALAD 90
- 11. BRIGHT DETOX SALAD 92
- 12. TASTY WARM POTATO SALAD 94
- 13. FRESH BROCCOLI SALAD FOR LUNCH 96

MAIN DISHES AND SIDE DISHES 98
- 14. DELICATE ALMOND SNACK 98
- 15. LAUNCH BURGERS WITH BACON AND PEACH 100
- 16. FAVORITE BBQ CHICKEN WITH A PEACHES 102
- 17. FANTASTIC HEALTHY LUNCH WITH SWEET FIGS 104
- 18. TENDER EASY DUCK CARNITAS 106
- 19. SWEET BROCCOLI WITH PINE NUTS 108
- 21. PICKLED "FRIED" GREEN TOMATOES WITH CREAMY-HERB SAUCE......112

SOUPS 114
- 22. RED VEGETABLE SOUP 114
- 23. NON-FAT DELICIOUS SOUP 116
- 24. DELIGHT BROWN RICE SOUP WITH LENTIL 118

HEALTHY TASTY SMOOTHIES 120

25. GREEN APPLE CIDER VINEGAR SMOOTHIE 120
26. SUNNY MANGO SMOOTHIE WITH APPLE CIDER VINEGAR 122
27. APPLE CIDER VINEGAR DETOX SMOOTHIE 124
28. MILKY BANANA SMOOTHIE WITH KALE 126
29. DELICIOUS ENERGY FRUIT SMOOTHIE.. 128

CONCLUSION **129**

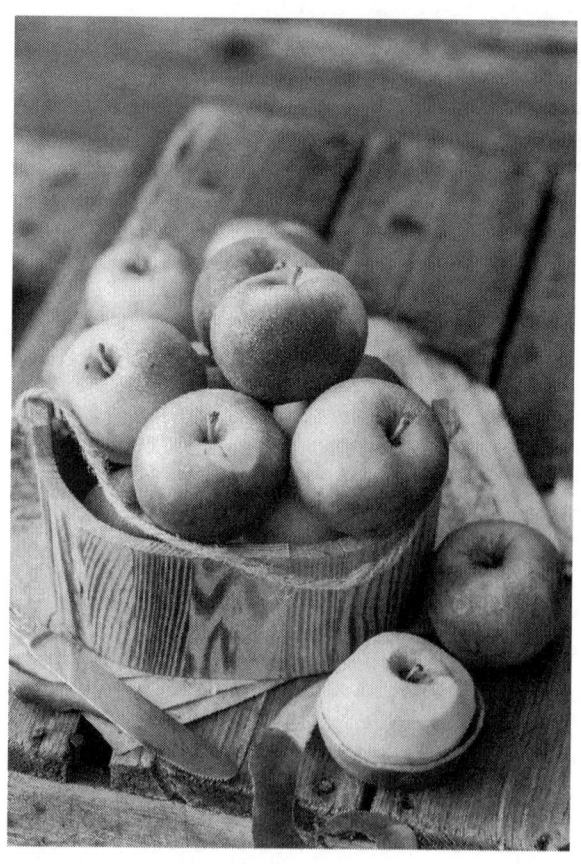

Introduction

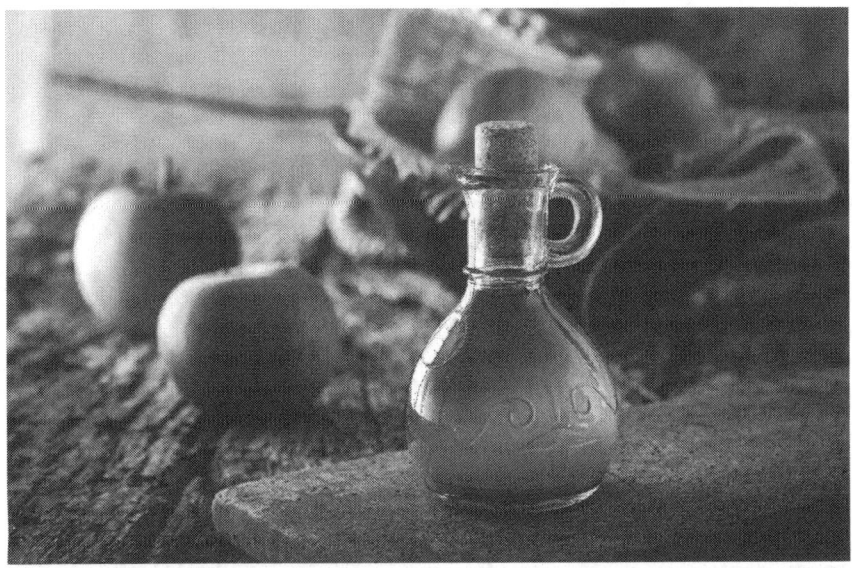

Like Salt, Apple Cider Vinegar changes the taste of everything. Let's admit it, this concoction doesn't have a great taste. In fact, no one would like to take a look at the faces they make while downing this drink.

Unless it's mixed with other drinks or incorporated into other foods, most people won't eat take it raw. However, all these seemingly downsides by far outweigh the endless possibilities that come with Apple Cider Vinegar.

Ever since the benefits of the Apple Cider Vinegar went viral, dieters are reawakening to the endless healing possibilities of this magical sour drink. This awakening has brought about an increase in the number of people seeking to stock this sour kitchen staple.

Apple Cider Vinegar is literally flying off the shelves at supermarkets!

If you have a bottle of apple cider vinegar in your pantry, then you can use it other than in the kitchen. Also known as ACV, this particular type of vinegar is made from apple must or cider. It has a medium amber color. It is commonly used in making marinades, salad dressings, chutney, or food preservatives. Apple cider vinegar undergoes fermentation process wherein the sugars are fermented and converted into acetic acid by a group of bacteria called Acetobacter. The acetic acid also gives the vinegar its unique sour taste.

The use of vinegar has been around since ancient times, and it was believed that Hippocrates used apple cider vinegar as a health tonic. On the other hand, apple cider vinegar is also a part of the first aid kit of soldiers in combat, and they use it to fight off scurvy, indigestion, and pneumonia.

The apple cider vinegar diet is one of the best diet regimes that are available today. What we know is that previous scientific literature indicates that apple cider vinegar is very effective in treating different conditions like diabetes and high blood pressure when taken in appropriate amounts. However, an excess of it can also lead to serious health repercussions like osteoporosis and esophageal burns. It is the reason why it is so important for people to use apple cider vinegar in appropriate amounts to get the most out of its health benefits.

There are many weight loss diets that you can do but the problem with most of the weight loss diets available today is that they require dieters to follow stringent rules and eat different kinds of foods each day. The problem with most weight loss diet programs is that it is hard to keep up with them for a long time. However, some weight loss diet programs do not require dieters to do a lot of things. One of the most enjoyable diet regimens that are very easy to follow is the apple cider vinegar diet.

Drinking apple cider vinegar has a lot of excellent benefits. However, drinking apple cider vinegar does not mean drinking a shot of pure apple cider vinegar. Learning how to drink apple cider vinegar properly is very important so that you can get the most benefits out of it.

Chapter 1: What Is Apple Cider Vinegar?

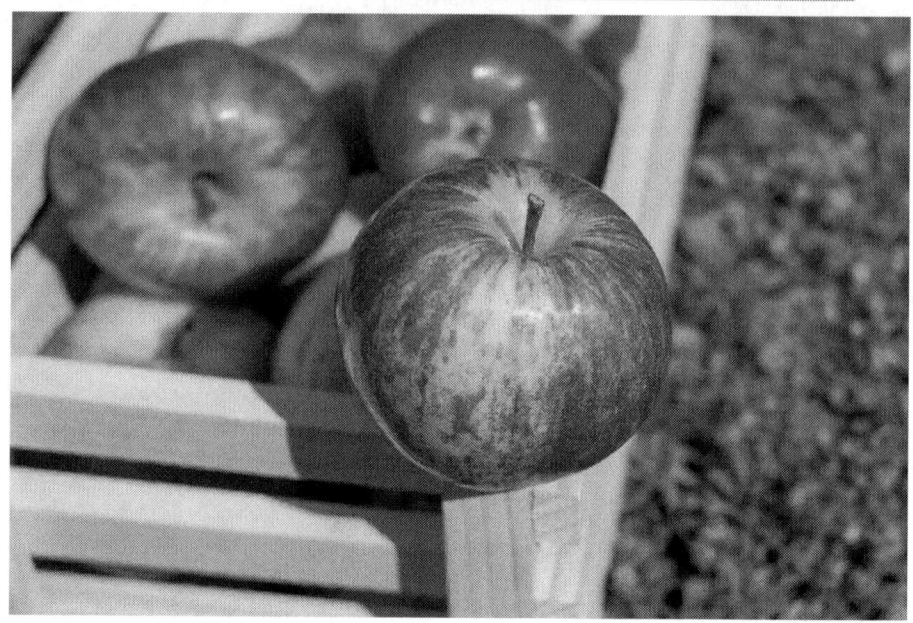

The word "vinegar" is a Latin word which means 'Sour Wine' and it has been used for its myriad of benefits that include but not limited to.

Apple Cider Vinegar (ACV) is the fermentation of high-quality apples.

The highest quality Apple Cider Vinegar is made from fresh, organic apples that are crushed into a must, and then, naturally aged in wooden or stainless-steel barrels. Apple cider vinegar undergoes a twostage fermentation process.

Stage 1: Apple Cider or Apple Wine comes from the first stage fermentation. This yeast fermentation is the same process that produces regular table wines like grapes that are fermented. A flavored ethanol alcohol produced in stage 1 is the stage that creates standard table wine.

Stage 2: As the mixture in Stage 1 continues, vinegar fermentation begins. The ethanol allowed to ferment further into this juncture produces acetic acid, also called vinegar. The quality of ingredients started in Stage 1 determines the quality of the finished product, whether it stops fermenting for alcohol in Stage 1 or stops in Stage 2 for vinegar.

When high quality, organic fresh apples are used, the 'mother' develops as part of the natural fermentation process. The mother is the strands floating within a cloudy amber liquid that are full of useful nutrients. Large business conglomerates filter out this dear mother leaving overly processed, commercial vinegar with a clear liquid. The mother gives a good part of the ACV its 'Apple Cider Vinegar Benefits' of health.

The non-organic and more highly commercialized ACV has the mother filtered out and pasteurized. Please don't use that for this book. Organic ACV, recommended here, contains the cloudy 'mother' and is not filtered or pasteurized. Favorite applications are in common foods around the world such as marinades, salad dressings, and even preservatives, but also in many more food products and methods than could ever be listed here.

Apple cider vinegar known for its nutritional and medicinal properties helps deal with many health issues. The simplest and ideal use of apple cider vinegar is by drinking 1 glass of clear water and 1 to 2 teaspoons of ACV. You can add some natural sweetener (honey, stevia). See below for an easy to sip drink you can enjoy 1 to 3 times each day. Get ready for a few nice health improvements no matter what your fitness level. Apple cider vinegar seems to be a great asset when used along with healthy eating choices and exercise.

Chapter 2: How to Make Apple Cider Vinegar

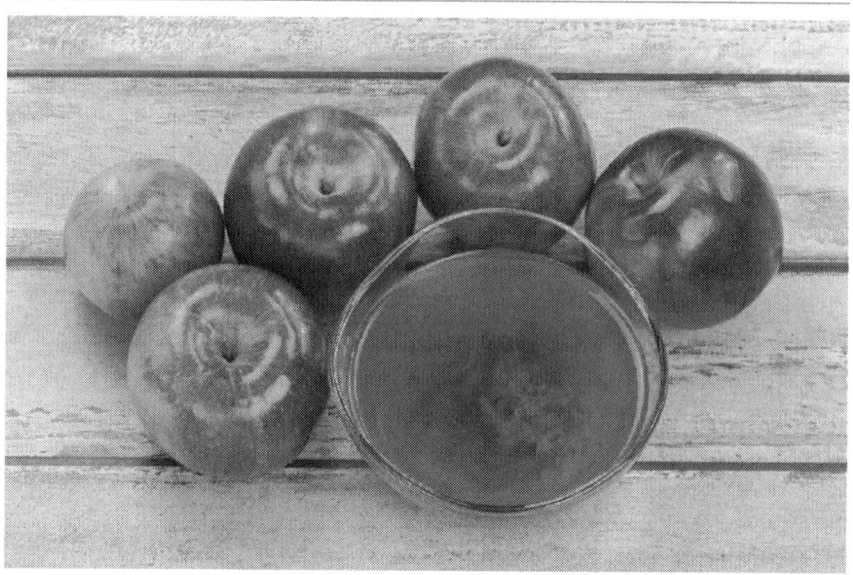

You can prepare apple cider vinegar in your own home. It's easy and way cheaper in comparison to market-bought ones.

What you need:

- Ten organic apples
- Water
- Cheesecloth
- One glass jar with wide mouth

How to do it:

1. Wash the apples thoroughly and allow them to dry.
2. Cut the apples into cubes. Include the peels and cores, but remove the stem.
3. Transfer the apple cubes into the glass jar and fill with water. Make sure to cover all the apples with water.

4. Keep it in a warm, dark place for about 2 to 3 weeks. You will start to notice scum on top of the liquid.
5. Strain the liquid and transfer back into the same glass container. Put it back into the same dark, warm area for another 4 to 6 weeks. Remember to stir the liquid every 2 to 3 days.
6. At week 4, taste the liquid if it is sour enough for you. If not, continue fermenting until your desired sourness is achieved.
7. Transfer to a glass bottle and enjoy it as you would.

Making your apple cider vinegar is easy. It does not require any special skills. It does require some patience since you have to wait for a few months before you can finally enjoy its benefits. Nonetheless, if you don't want to wait that long, you can always buy in the market. Just make sure to choose the one that still contains the mother to enjoy its maximum benefits.

Chapter 3: Tips When Making and using Apple Cider Vinegar

Always use sterilized glass jar for fermenting and storing. Before fermenting, ensure that there are no soap residues or debris left in the bottle as it will affect the quality and taste of your ACV. Your cheesecloth should also be clean and dry.

Remember, when the scum that forms on top of your mixture is white, then that means that it's good. However, if it is a different color other than white (black, blue, green or gray), then you have to discard it. It means bad bacteria has infested your ferment and it can be harmful to your health if you consume it.

If you have leftover apple peels and core, do not throw them. You can ferment them instead and turn them into apple cider. If possible, use organic apples to minimize your risk of ingesting pesticides used in commercially grown apples.

Apple Cider Vinegar is getting famous for its extensive uses and benefits in the health component, but like everything else, too much consumption of anything does lead to some problems.

Following are the few side effects of Apple Cider Vinegar if taken in large amount.

- Those patients who have type 1 diabetes, ACV may reduce the digestion process which in turns, might worsen the gastro paresis symptoms and blood sugar level might be difficult to control
- Apple cider vinegar contains acids, which if taken with juices that already have acids, might worsen

the situation and the person might feel dizzy and nausea

- There is increased amount of acetic acid in ACV, which might lead to the teeth damage and decay
- If given to children, apple cider vinegar might hurt or burn the throat. There was a woman whose throat was burnt because the ACV pill got stuck in her esophagus
- Many people reported that they applied apple cider vinegar as a treatment for skin moles or acne, and then their skin got burned by using too much of it
- It is very dangerous to take apple cider vinegar if you are using medication for your diabetes or heart diseases
- By detoxifying the body through ACV, there is a possibility that people might get headaches or migraines. When the body is detoxifying, brain stimulates toxins which are healthy but also very painful
- If you are experiencing extreme itching after using apple cider vinegar for few days, this may be a sign of some allergic reaction. Stop taking ACV immediately until the itching goes away
- Due to the high acetic acid, ACV causes potassium to be of low levels in the blood, causing hypokalemia. Because low levels of potassium, a person might feel dizziness, nausea, excessive urination, cramps, *etc.*
- Those who have osteoporosis should avoid taking apple cider vinegar altogether as it can reduce the density of bone minerals, meaning, it can make bones weak

Nevertheless, going by the little scientific evidence that is available, ACV is definitely useful and a good candidate worth pondering about. At the very least, it is outright safe. No detrimental side effects have been recorded with **NORMAL CONSUMPTION**. One of the best ways to consume it is incorporating it in your drinks or in your cooking. A widely accepted dosage ranges between 1-3 teaspoons per day. This may come in form of diluting it in water or even using it as a dressing for your food. Don't get it twisted, though going above that may be considered excessive consumption and may be rewarded with disastrous tidings.

There are more benefits to ACV than the side effects, but special precautions should be taken while drinking it. Take small dosages of ACV and try to avoid its exposure with teeth. And after you have drunk it, wash your mouth properly.

Chapter 4: Apple Cider Vinegar Benefits

It's well understood that vinegar is a product of fermentation and therefore apple cider vinegar comes from the fermentation of crushed apples. Although apple cider vinegar has been used extensively in the ancient times, it wasn't until 1958 when apple cider vinegar was first studied. This product has been promoted as an alternative medicine which has been critical in treating various ailments since as far back as the 1950s. It has been acknowledged by well-known researchers like D.C. Jarvis that ACV can treat a wide variety of diseases like easing pain and aches. Jarvis conducted extensive research on the benefits of using apple cider vinegar and has documented them in his books.

In the book of Dr. D.C. Jarvis entitled Folk Medicine: A Vermont Doctor's Guide to Good Health, Dr. Jarvis recommended that apple cider vinegar as an all-cure medicine for different maladies. In his book, Dr. Jarvis also noted that apple cider vinegar could also be enhanced with honey.

The fascinating thing about this product is its ability to remain natural even after fermentation due to the retaining of its nutritional characteristics and gaining, even more, qualities due to the enzymes and other acids formed during fermentation. It cumulatively gives apple cider vinegar more health benefits than your everyday apple. It is an amazing, low-cost medicine for a multitude of common and complex ailments.

The benefits of apple cider vinegar include enhancing weight loss, with studies indicating that a bread meal spiced up by the vinegar creates a more satisfying and fuller feeling. Apple cider vinegar helps in stabilizing blood sugar longer, which assists in controlling appetite, actually reducing the amount of food you would eat. By controlling blood sugar levels, it can reduce the effects and chances of diabetes occurring in humans.

HELPS TO REGULATE BLOOD SUGAR

With the number of people suffering diabetes in the US expected to double by 2050, researchers are looking to harness the benefits of ACV.

According to a research conducted by Arizona University, evidence supports that ACV helps improve insulin sensitivity to people suffering from diabetes. In particular, those with type-2 diabetes, it has been shown that it reduces postprandial glycemia and increases satiety. These two are metabolic effects that may prove useful for people struggling with diabetes.

By drinking 20 grams of this sour drink before eating meals with high starch content, you greatly reduce insulin fluctuation and sugar levels.

REDUCES CHOLESTEROL AND TRIGLYCERIDE LEVELS

Cholesterol and triglyceride are BF that continually circulates within our bodies. They are both useful and harmful. Our bodies require them to function. However, in large quantities they are harmful.

According to a research conducted in rats by the University of Shizoku in Japan in collaboration with Mizkan Corporation, the acetic acid that is found In ACV greatly helped reduce the cholesterol and triglyceride levels when it was consumed together with food that contained high cholesterol levels.

And since this research was done on animals, it has not been proven that this would resonate with human beings.

Another research by Babol University in Iran suggests that the Apple Cider Vinegar can be used to prevent heart problems and atherosclerosis.

PROMOTES WEIGHT LOSS

According to another Study by Mizkhan Group Corporation individuals who took a daily dose of ACV showed significant body fat loss compared to those who did not. The study went further ahead to establish that since high sugar levels in your body make you hungrier, the ACV is able to lower the sugar level preventing you from packing those unwanted calories.

FIGHTS CANCER

Cancer has turned out to be a silent killer that manifests in advance stages when little can be done to counter it or even cure it.

In the 2014 more than 1.6 million people in the United States were diagnosed with cancer while more than half a million succumbed to the same.

According to a Study by University of Crete in Greece, vinegar has shown that it can greatly help shrink cancer cells. And although the tests were done on lab animals, scientists believe the same can be replicated to human beings.

On the other side of the world in China, researchers have shown that incorporating ACV to vegetable recipes can greatly reduce esophageal cancer.

STIMULATES DIGESTION AND MINERAL ABSORPTION

Apple Cider Vinegar is a rich source of vitamin B and C. Additionally; it also contains Acetic which is a compound Acid which is paramount in escalating mineral absorption in our bodies. With the help that Apple Cider Vinegar provides in the digestion of food, it is considered in all health and nutrition related food recipes.

UTILIZATION OF IRON
Apple Cider Vinegar improves iron utilization by your body. Iron is a major component that helps your body to transport oxygen to the body cells. It's this attribute of the ACV that helps the body to utilize energy making it ideal for people seeking to lose weight.

GREAT SOURCE OF POTASSIUM
If taken on a regular basis, ACV will supply your body with an endless dose of Potassium (73 mg/100g of ACV). This in return ensures a balanced dose of potassium to your body and your diet.

PROMOTES HEALTHY DETOXIFICATION
Apple cider vinegar helps in cleansing the lymph node and body mucus. This facilitates better circulation. When your circulation works optimally, your body is able to get rid of toxins and improve your immune system.

➢ EASY TO USE
Apple cider vinegar can be prepared as a salad dressing very quickly, diluted with hot or cold water, or added to hot water with a little honey or stevia and taken as a tea. It also can control indigestion of certain foods by clearing chronic acid when the two are combined.

Despite the enormous capabilities of apple cider vinegar as a medicine, especially by patients suffering from diabetes and heart diseases, it should always first be approved by health providers as it can interact with laxatives and diuretics. This interaction may be problematic.

ACV is also a great ingredient in Seafood, meat and Veg food. Adding a few spoonfuls into your food or drinks are some of the other ways you can use ACV for your Lunch or Dinner recipes.

➢ SKIN CARE

Apple cider vinegar can be applied to the skin to control ailments such as acne and discolorations of the skin. The major component of apple cider vinegar is acetic acid meaning that the product is harsh and therefore should be diluted with water before use. Otherwise, it may cause contact burns to the skin or damage tissues in the throat.

TONE YOUR SKIN

If you're one of the many people who spend a pretty penny on top-of-the-line skin toners, you may be relieved to hear that you can instead use apple cider vinegar! When it comes to skin treatments, the same elements that make ACV effective in treating overall health conditions make it an excellent product for treating diseases of the skin as well. The purpose of a skin toner is to remove dead skin cells and oil, refreshing the area of the face and revealing a rejuvenated layer of skin that appears clean, bright, and supple. ACV's vitamins and naturally occurring acids are a safe and efficient manner to improve the look and feel of skin while also restoring the natural balance of oils and pH of the skin.

Specifically, the acetic and malic acids contained within apple cider vinegar improve the health and appearance of the skin by:

- Gently removing dead skin cells
- Balancing the pH levels of the skin
- Removing dirt and oils from the pores

- Treating the causes of acne and unsightly blemishes
- Providing vitamin C–based antioxidant benefits to restore skin cell health and reverse oxidative damage

TO MAKE A SKIN TONER, COMBINE:

1/2 cup warm water • 1/3 cup ACV

Soak a cotton ball in the solution and apply directly to the skin of the face and neck. The remaining mixture can be stored in a dark, cool place in an airtight container.

CLEANSE YOUR PORES

Your face is exposed to some toxins throughout the day. Airborne elements and visible dirt and grime adversely affect the appearance and health of your skin. While environmental factors are to blame to an extent, the more common contributor to clogged pores is touching your face with your hands—which you likely do dozens of times per day, consciously or subconsciously. When your pores become clogged with unhealthy deposits from your hands, the skin is unable to "breathe" and can develop an oily, greasy, or excessively dry condition.

Many cleansers on the market contain harsh or abrasive components that can aggravate the skin's natural balance of oils and pH, and lead to unhealthy or uncomfortable skin conditions. As a natural alternative to chemical-laden products, apple cider vinegar provides cleansing properties that rid the skin of harmful deposits and keep the skin's pores open and healthy. By restoring the natural pH balance of the skin, ACV has also shown to regulate the oils produced by the skin, resulting in a healthier balance of oil production and minimizing the clogging of pores.

TO MAKE A PORE CLEANSER, COMBINE IN A BOWL:

1/2 cup warm water • 1/2 cup ACV

Use a facecloth to absorb the liquid, ring out the excess, and gently rub the skin with the towel. Repeatedly rinse and reabsorb the ACV mixture, reapplying the mixture to the skin until the skin looks and feels refreshed and bright.

EASE A SUNBURN

When the skin is exposed to excessive sunlight, with or without sunblock, the irritation that results is not only uncomfortable and unsightly, but it can be downright dangerous! More and more research directly associates sun exposure to unhealthy or even cancerous growth of the skin cells. If you've got a sunburn, the most efficient way to soothe and repair the skin is to apply natural restorative elements that aid in the regeneration and repair of the skin's cells. One of the most useful agents in improving cell health is vitamin C, and many products on the market that claim to improve skin health contain this essential vitamin. While the cosmetic products available temporarily relieve sunburns or improve the look and feel of skin, few include the combination of elements provided by apple cider vinegar that can improve skin health safely, naturally, and effectively.

Through its strong acids and enzymes that restore the natural balance of the naturally occurring oils produced by the skin, ACV alleviates the tightening and burning sensations resulting from a sunburn. Replenishing the vitamin C stores on-site, topical use of ACV also aids in the cell regeneration in the skin while preventing free radical damage that can cause cancerous cell changes.

TO MAKE A SKIN SOAK, COMBINE:

1/2 cup lukewarm water • 1/2 cup ACV

Apply the ACV mixture directly to the skin with a moist towel or sponge.

TO MAKE A SOOTHING SOAK, COMBINE:

Tub full of water • 2 cups ACV

Soak for 30 minutes.

TO MAKE A DRINK, COMBINE:

1 cup water or freshly squeezed orange juice • one tablespoon aloe vera juice, organic • one tablespoon ACV

Drink up to three times daily.

By combining these three treatments, you can alleviate the symptoms that result from a sunburn and actually treat cell damage that resulted from the sun exposure.

MINIMIZE PSORIASIS

Psoriasis is an uncomfortable and unsightly condition that is thought to be caused by trauma to the skin, stress, smoking, excessive alcohol consumption, sun exposure, and certain medications. Characterized by bright or red patches of skin that may or may not itch, psoriasis is a non-contagious condition resulting from the body's autoimmune system seeing the skin cells as pathogens and over-stimulating the production of skin cells. While many over-the-counter creams can provide relief of psoriasis and treat the skin condition, many contain harsh chemicals or produce undesirable side effects that can further irritate the skin. Lifestyle changes that minimize the factors that are assumed to contribute to the condition (such as quitting smoking and reducing alcohol consumption, sun exposure, and stress) will help improve the effectiveness of any psoriasis treatment.

Apple cider vinegar has become a notable treatment for skin conditions like psoriasis because of the multitude of beneficial elements it can provide internally, as well as to the site of irritation. ACV contains:

- Immunity-boosting vitamin C
- Blood-quality-improving enzymes
- Reparative antioxidant properties

Apple cider vinegar is a natural product that can improve the health of your skin while also maintaining proper functioning of the body's systems that directly support the skin's health.

TO MAKE A TOPICAL TREATMENT, COMBINE:

1/2 cup water • 1/2 cup ACV

Soak a towel in the solution and apply it directly to the affected area for 30 minutes.

TO MAKE A DRINK THAT SUPPORTS OVERALL SKIN HEALTH, COMBINE:

1 cup water • one tablespoon ACV

Drink daily.

REDUCE THE APPEARANCE OF FACIAL "MASKS."

Using a combination of apple cider vinegar and other health-restoring items as a topical facial mask has shown to alleviate symptoms of skin irritation like redness, acne, and discoloration while improving the appearance and quality of the skin. Helping to balance the natural oil production of the skin on the face and neck, apple cider vinegar's acetic and malic acids assist in unclogging pores and removing grime that can be deposited on the face throughout everyday life. Helping to restore a beneficial pH balance to the skin, ACV has shown drastic results in acne sufferers' reduction of irritation and incidence of pimples and blemishes on the skin. Rich in vitamin C and beta carotene, ACV's most impressive benefit is the reduction in free radical damage to the skin on a cellular level, improving the health of the skin and preventing further skin damage that can result from exposure to everyday toxins like smoke, UV light, and air pollution.

TO MAKE A BENEFICIAL SKIN MASK, MASH THE FOLLOWING INGREDIENTS INTO A PASTE:

1/2 cup ACV • 1/2 of 1 avocado • one tablespoon natural, unprocessed, organic honey

Apply directly to the skin for 15–30 minutes, removing the mask by rinsing with warm water.

This particular combination of foods contains abundant amounts of antioxidants, healthy fats, vitamins, minerals, and enzymes that absorb into the skin and help to:

- Promote blood flow
- Repair damage
- Restore skin health
- Regulate pH and oil production
- Remove dirt and germs from the skin's surface and pores

➤ HAIR CARE

Apple cider vinegar can help maintain soft hair especially from the use of conditioners and styling products due to the presence of acetic acid within the vinegar. It can also maintain proper hair pH, control dandruff, and kill bacteria. Even the smallest benefits of this miracle vinegar are great!

Do you spend countless hours and dollars on your regular hair regimen? Do you find yourself dealing with unruly locks that lack the volume, shine, or length you dream of? Are you finding it harder and harder to maintain your hair's natural beauty? Or are you simply tired of wasting money on chemical-laden hair-care products that promise the world but fail to deliver? If you consider how many hair products you use on a daily basis, between shampooing and styling, you can imagine how much residue from those products gets left behind. All of that residue and buildup from the products that are intended to help your hair result hinder natural growth, shine, body, highlights, and so much more! Because of the damage, this buildup can cause to your hair's follicles, cuticles, pores, and ends; you can be left with an unmanageable head of hair that is so unhealthy no product could help! Look no further: apple cider vinegar will restore natural health to your hair and help you attain the hair you've always dreamed of!

ACV contains an astounding variety of naturally occurring acids, enzymes, vitamins, and minerals that work synergistically to deliver healthy nutrition hair requires, can be used in different formulations to act as everything from a clarifying rinse and shampoo to an adequate preparation for more vibrant and longer-lasting color-treatments and is safe enough to drink.

Supported with scientific explanations of how and why this product and the combinations and treatments for each particular benefit work to eliminate the hair issues you deal with daily, these easy-to-create and simple-to-use treatments can quickly provide the results you want while repairing the damage that your hair "care" products have done.

The bottom line is this: If you want to achieve the results you have dreamt of for ages, are tired of spending time and money on products and treatments that are not delivering, and want to use an all-natural product, try apple cider vinegar. Start repairing your hair and get on your way to the beautiful hair you imagine by implementing these ACV treatments today!

HELP THINNING HAIR

Thinning hair can be an embarrassing condition, and it doesn't only strike older men. Women of all ages are becoming a large part of the consumer pool looking for remedies to prevent thinning hair. While prescription drugs and over-the-counter medications promise to deliver robust results, they often contain harsh chemicals and additives that can pose health risks and aggravate certain medical conditions. If you're looking to reap the benefits of thinning hair treatments safely and more efficiently with natural products, look no further than a good bottle of apple cider vinegar.

By applying apple cider vinegar directly to the site of thinning hair, you can:

- Improve the blood circulation of the scalp
- Improve the blood flow to hair follicles
- Ensure efficient delivery of essential nutrients to the scalp

These health-boosting benefits provided by ACV help to promote hair growth and prevent hair loss. ACV also contains valuable vitamins, minerals, and proteins that provide the skin with essential nutrients needed to produce healthy hair and maintain quality proteins within the hair shaft.

TO MAKE A HAIR TONIC, COMBINE:

Two tablespoons ACV • 1 tablespoon water • 1/2 teaspoon cayenne pepper

Apply directly to the site of thinning hair, rubbing the mixture into the scalp for 5 minutes. Allow it to sit on the scalp for 1 hour before shampooing as usual. You can start to see results within 2–4 weeks.

Two chemical compounds in cayenne, "capsaicin", and "quercetin", are the beneficial components that help stimulate hair growth by stimulating hair follicles and improving blood flow to the scalp.

BEAT DANDRUFF

Dandruff can be caused by some factors but is most likely due to:

- Chemicals within certain hair-care products
- Specific types of bacteria that affect the scalp
- Toxic elements in the environment

Regardless of the cause, apple cider vinegar can restore the natural pH balance to the scalp, moisturize the skin, and return the hair condition to one without dry, flaky, or irritating residue.

ACV provides essential acids that act for returning the scalp's pH to a normal, healthy level, which is also beneficial to the balance of oils needed to maintain moisture without an overly oily residue. ACV is also able to provide relief to the scalp by reducing inflammation, improving circulation beneath the skin of the scalp, and delivering essential nutrients directly to the sites affected.

<u>TO MAKE An SCALP-SOOTHING SOLUTION, COMBINE:</u>

1/2 cup ACV • 1 cup warmed liquid coconut oil

Apply the mixture to the scalp, and allow to sit on the scalp for 30–45 minutes. Rinse before shampooing and conditioning as normal.

You can also follow up the ACV and coconut oil treatment with this scalp rinse.

TO MAKE A SCALP RINSE, COMBINE:

1/3 cup ACV • 1 cup warm water

Rinse the scalp with the solution after shampooing and conditioning, before towel-drying hair.

MAKE YOUR HAIR RINSE

While most hair-care products efficiently provide what they promise, many leave unsightly residue and buildup on the hair follicles, hair shafts, and scalp. This buildup can lead to excessively oily hair, unmanageable frizz, or dark color. Comically, many hair products promise to remove this residue by using chemicals and harsh abrasives that can lead to hair that is dry and unmanageable, meaning you traded one problem for another. By using apple cider vinegar as a rinse following the usual shampooing and conditioning treatments, you can actually remove residue and restore your hair's health, shine, and color naturally and without adverse side effects.

With acids and enzymes that cleanse and vitamins and minerals that nourish, apple cider vinegar can clear the hair of debris and buildup without damaging the hair's follicles or disrupt the scalp's pH balance.

TO MAKE A HAIR RINSE, COMBINE:

1 cup water • 1/2 cup ACV

Apply it to the hair following your routine of shampooing and conditioning. Allow the mixture to sit on the hair and scalp for 5 minutes before rinsing with warm water. Repeating this procedure with every other wash will ensure your hair stays free of buildup that weighs down hair.

MAKE YOUR SHAMPOO

Some shampoos leave you with luscious locks that bounce, shine, and stay frizz-free, while others leave your hair feeling weighed down, dried out, or full of frizz. Trying out different brands can be costly, time-consuming, and damaging to your hair. By using apple cider vinegar as a shampoo alternative, you can naturally cleanse the hair and add beauty and health to your strands. You might even see and feel an improvement in the quality of your hair after just one treatment! ACV is inexpensive, natural, and doesn't contain harsh chemicals and additions (which can increase the frequency of bad hair days). ACV will supply your hair with these amazing benefits:

- Cleanse your hair of grime and build up
- Add health-fortifying vitamins and minerals directly to the hair and scalp for improved shine, volume, and bounce
- Provide everything from restorative proteins to pH-neutralizing enzymes
- Promote hair health and restore beauty to strands
- Gently remove environmental deposits

<u>TO MAKE SHAMPOO, COMBINE IN A BOTTLE:</u>

1/2 cup ACV • 2 tablespoons lemon juice • 1 cup water

Use the mixture in place of your shampoo, massaging it into the scalp and strands, rinsing, and proceeding to the condition as you routinely would. You can use this shampoo substitute every wash, or use it alternately with your regular shampoo.

MAKE YOUR CONDITIONER

Nowadays, you can find deep conditioning treatments at home and in the salon, as well as balms and solutions that promise to leave hair silky and hydrated. The variety of conditioning treatments is dizzying. Depending upon whether your hair is oily, dry, curly, or straight, different conditioners designed to treat all hair types may fall flat on delivering their promised results. Surprisingly enough, the same bottle of apple cider vinegar you use for your daily tonics that keep you healthy and energized can also work wonders as a conditioner for hair of all types, shades, and textures. Some treatment options may be available, but few provide the nutrients contained in ACV, are as inexpensive as ACV, and provide results after the very first treatment as ACV does!

Combined with the additional conditioning components of coconut oil, ACV is an effective conditioner that tames frizz, fights tangles, and keeps locks lustrous while improving the pH levels of the scalp and closing the hair follicles.

TO MAKE CONDITIONER, COMBINE IN A BOTTLE:

1/2 cup ACV • 1/4 cup liquid coconut oil • 1 cup water

Apply the treatment to your hair, cover hair with a shower cap, and allow the mixture to sit for 30 minutes. Then rinse and dry, revealing renewed hair with restored health.

COMBAT BALDNESS

Alopecia can occur as a result of genetics, repeated damaging hair treatments, or lack of sufficient dietary elements that support the health and growth of hair. In its unfiltered state, ACV contains some important enzymes, proteins, vitamins, minerals, and naturally occurring acids that combine to:

- Contribute cleansing and restorative elements directly to the site of baldness
- Remove agitating causes that can contribute to baldness
- Improve the conditions of the hair and scalp, promoting new hair growth and maintaining the health of that hair growth

Chemical-laden hair-regenerating products can irritate the scalp, damage the hair, and interfere with the absorption and utilization of essential elements needed for healthy hair growth. Instead, use only natural-ingredient shampoos, conditioners, and treatments such as ACV. Finally, to spot-treat baldness and internally balance essential physical nutrients, you can use two effective treatments: a topical ACV treatment and an ingested ACV tonic.

TO MAKE A TONIC, COMBINE:

1/2 cup water • 1/2 cup ACV • 1/2 teaspoon cayenne pepper

Apply the mixture directly to the scalp at the areas where baldness is appearing. Leave the mixture on the scalp for 30 minutes, then shampoo and condition as normal. Following this routine on a daily basis has shown to improve baldness in 2–4 weeks!

TO MAKE A DRINKABLE TONIC, COMBINE:

1 cup water • one tablespoon ACV

Drink daily.

This drink provides the dietary components in ACV such as the vitamins, minerals, enzymes, and acids that:

- Support the health of systems directly related to the growth and health of hair, such as metabolism and blood flow
- Help resolve deficiencies that can contribute to baldness, such as some B vitamins, vitamin C, vitamin D, and iron

IMPROVE HAIR POROSITY

"Porosity" is the term that refers to the hair's ability to absorb and retain moisture. Low-porosity hair can absorb and retain moisture well, while high-porosity hair does not. The strands of your hair contain pores and hair shafts that allow moisture into the hair when wet. When you are suffering from dry, oily, frizzy, or unmanageable hair, it is most commonly due to damage to the hair's cuticle and pores, complicating the process of the hair's ability to obtain and retain moisture. The hair's cuticle is the outer layer of the hair that looks very similar to shingles on a roof, and when grime from the environment or some styling products and processes settle on the hair's cuticles, it can result in clogged pores that don't allow moisture to be absorbed. The hair's pores can also be affected by styling processes that damage the cuticle. As a result, the pores do not open to allow moisture in; nor do they close tightly (which is what allows the hair to appear shiny and sleek, without frizz). When these standard processes are troubled by damaging products and treatments, the effective corrective treatment has to focus on restoring the natural health to the hair's porosity. For an effective, natural solution for high-porosity hair, you can use apple cider vinegar.

By combining natural ingredients that contain protein, fats, and vitamins and minerals, you can deliver essential elements to your hair that restore hair health quickly, easily, and naturally!

<u>TO MAKE An HAIR-CARE SOLUTION, COMBINE IN A BLENDER AT ROOM TEMPERATURE:</u>

1/2 cup ACV • 1/2 cup almond milk • 1/4 cup liquid coconut oil • two tablespoons honey

Apply to the hair. Once the hair is soaked with the ACV treatment, put on a shower cap, and leave on for 30 minutes before rinsing. Performing this treatment every day or every other day, you will notice a return of healthy shine and texture to your hair in 1–2 weeks.

DETANGLE HAIR

When your hair is a tangled mess, and you have trouble simply brushing or combing it after a shower, you may be inclined to use a detangling product. While many products on the market promise to leave your hair healthy and free of tangles, a significant number of them contain chemicals or unnatural substances that can strip right elements from hair, leaving your strands lackluster and damaged. To fight tangles while retaining the health of hair, try ACV!

Containing restorative and essential vitamins and minerals, ACV can reduce tangles by removing residue and buildup left behind from cleaning products, while also moisturizing and conditioning your strands and making them more manageable and easier to style.

<u>TO MAKE A DETANGLING SPRAY, COMBINE IN A SPRAY BOTTLE:</u>

½ cup ACV • 1 cup water

Spray your hair with the ACV solution from the scalp to the ends of your hair, combing through locks and relieving tangles. There's no need to rinse the solution, so you can only style your hair as you normally would and enjoy the added benefits of shine and manageability, too!

REDUCE FRIZZ

Frizzy hair is a frustrating condition that can be caused by the weather or extensive exposure to damaging elements contained in hair products and hair treatments. The crux of frizzy hair issues is high porosity that is due by the shaft of hair strands remaining open and unable to retain moisture. The drying out of these strands makes them susceptible to effects of the climate or styling products and treatments that lead to hair appearing "frizzy." By delivering naturally therapeutic proteins and nutrients to your hair strands, you can spot-treat frizziness and enjoy healthy, shiny, manageable hair. You might see "natural" products on the market, but be sure you read the ingredients carefully—many are labeled "natural", but they still contain certain preservatives or synthetic materials that can lead to hair damage. To avoid unnecessary "bad hair days" caused by frizz, you need to look no further than apple cider vinegar.

ACV contains plentiful amounts of proteins and enzymes that provide hair with therapeutic health benefits.

<u>TO MAKE AN IN-SHOWER ANTIFRIZZ TREATMENT, COMBINE IN A BOTTLE:</u>

½ cup ACV • ½ cup water • 2 teaspoons liquid coconut oil

After conditioning in the shower, apply the mixture to your hair and leave it on for 5 minutes. Then rinse the solution from the hair and dry as you would routinely.

<u>TO MAKE A PRESTYLING, FRIZZ-FIGHTING SOLUTION, COMBINE IN A SPRAY BOTTLE:</u>

1 cup water • 1/2 cup ACV

Saturate damp hair with the ACV spray. After allowing the spray to settle for 5 minutes, towel-dry and style as you would routinely.

PREVENT SPLIT ENDS

Split ends occur when the end of a hair strand breaks into two strands that then proceed to divide the hair from the bottom up. Not only does this damage the hair, but it can make the appearance and the maintenance and styling of hair confusing and frustrating. By trimming only the ends of your hair every month, you can prevent split ends before they start and keep healthy hair free of split-end damage. Another way to prevent split ends is to ensure that you have the proper intake of essential vitamins and minerals that contribute to healthy hair growth, like silica, calcium, vitamin C, and B vitamins. A full vitamin and mineral intake will improve your hair's health from the inside out and prevent split ends from occurring. To treat split ends most effectively, you can use all-natural, unfiltered, organic apple cider vinegar as an ingested preventive measure as well as a topical remedy, providing relief from split ends forever!

<u>TO MAKE A DRINK THAT ENSURES YOUR VITAMIN AND MINERAL INTAKE IS OPTIMAL, COMBINE:</u>

1 cup water • one tablespoon ACV

Drink daily.

TO MAKE A TOPICAL TREATMENT FOR SPLIT ENDS, COMBINE:

1/2 cup water • 1/2 cup ACV • 1/4 cup mashed avocado

Rub the mixture into the bottom 1/4 of hair, and allow to sit for 30 minutes before rinsing thoroughly. Repeat this treatment two or three times weekly, and you can actually prevent split ends, seeing results in a matter of a few short weeks.

KILL AND PREVENT HEAD LICE

Head lice can be an embarrassing and frustrating issue, especially considering that the most commonly affected population is school-aged children. In close quarters like classrooms with large numbers of children, head lice are easily transferred from person to person. Limiting exposure to anyone with confirmed head lice is the first preventive measure that can actually reduce the chance of contracting head lice. If you find yourself dealing with a confirmed case of head lice, though, you must not only treat the head lice but also take precautionary measures to ensure the insects die and have no chance of returning to cause the condition again.

Many drugstore products are available that can treat head lice, but most contain chemicals and synthetic additives that can be hazardous to your health or dangerous to adults and children with particular skin sensitivities. As a natural alternative, try ACV.

TO MAKE A HEAD LICE TREATMENT:

Apply undiluted apple cider vinegar to the hair and scalp, covering the hair with a shower cap. Allow the vinegar to remain on the hair for at least 4–5 hours. After removing the cap and rinsing the hair with water, carefully comb through the hair with a fine-tooth comb, eliminating the nits and eggs.

Repeat this process daily until all lice and eggs are gone.

PROMOTE HAIR GROWTH

The number of hair-growth products on the market is overwhelmingly large and is increasing every year. The difference between one product and another can be the chemical components, the claims to be "all-natural," or the guarantees that growth will follow the product's use. While the promotions can seem promising, the actual results can vary product to product and person to person depending on some factors. By combining some practical hair-growth methods with ACV, you can efficiently and inexpensively improve your hair growth naturally.

Apple cider vinegar has long been promoted for an enormous number of uses that promote health because of its high amounts of essential vitamins and minerals. With natural acids, enzymes, and proteins also contained within every drop of ACV; it is now accepted as an effective ingredient for treating hair loss and supporting hair growth. By massaging the scalp daily, eating a balanced diet high in protein, and minimizing the hair's exposure to heat treatments and harmful chemicals, you can maintain hair health.

<u>TO MAKE A NIGHTLY HAIR GROWTH TREATMENT, COMBINE:</u>

1 cup ACV • 1 cup aloe juice

Apply directly to the scalp and throughout the hair to the ends, cover with a shower cap, and sleep with the used mixture on the hair for 7–8 hours. A shower or rinse your hair in the morning. You can improve the health of your hair, restore natural essential nutrients, and see and feel the results in 2–4 weeks.

ADD SHINE

One of the most common complaints about hair is that it is dull, and hair-care companies know this all too well. To the rescue of dull hair, millions of products that promise to return the light-reflective shine to your dark mane are available at your favorite grocery store, drugstore, salon, or hair product website and can range in price from $1 to over $100! If you're hoping to remedy your lackluster locks and return the beautiful glow we associate with healthy hair, you needn't look any further than your trusty bottle of apple cider vinegar.

By introducing apple cider vinegar into your diet and hair treatment routine, you can:

- Restore the natural balance of nutrients to your body's systems that promote hair health
- Topically improve your hair's condition and appearance by stripping away residue and build-up left behind from styling products
- Repair damage done by heat and chemical treatments intended to style, color, or treat hair

TO MAKE An SHINY-HAIR DRINK, COMBINE:

1 cup water • one tablespoon ACV

Drink daily to deliver an abundance of vitamins, minerals, acids, and enzymes that assist in maintaining hair health.

TO MAKE A TOPICAL HAIR SOLUTION, COMBINE:

1 cup water • 1 cup ACV • 2 tablespoons essential oil of peppermint

After shampooing and conditioning, apply the solution to hair and work through strands. Allow the mixture to sit for 5–10 minutes before rinsing thoroughly.

This treatment can restore hair health to the shaft, pores, and cuticles of hair strands, helping to repair damage and restore a healthy sheen naturally.

PROMOTE SCALP HEALTH

ACV is an alternative to expensive, synthetic products that may or may not work to make your scalp healthier. It's a quick and inexpensive, all-natural, nutrient-rich option, whether your issue with scalp health is mild or severe.

The health of your scalp directly affects the quality of your day. If that sounds a bit extreme, speak to someone who suffers from severe dandruff, bouts of baldness or hair loss, or frequent itchy scalp, and you'll find that scalp health is serious business. By walking into any hair-care aisle of almost any store, you can see that scalp health is also a lucrative business, with thousands of products designed to restore health to your scalp for a price. Whether you pay that price at the expense of the product, or by suffering from health conditions that can be aggravated or a direct result of the chemicals or synthetic ingredients contained in the product, many of the scalp-restorative products don't live up to their promises or are far more than you bargained for.

TO RESTORE HEALTH TO YOUR SCALP, COMBINE:

1 cup water • 1/2 cup ACV • 1 teaspoon cayenne pepper • one teaspoon organic honey

Wet hair and apply the mixture to scalp, rubbing into scalp thoroughly. Allow mixture to set on hair and scalp for 30 minutes before rinsing, shampooing, and conditioning as usual. Repeat daily or weekly.

➢ STRESS & ODOR

Conditions of stress and tiredness can be cured by apple cider vinegar which counteracts lactic acid build up by stress. It contains enzymes and potassium which are responsible for relieving fatigue.

Apple cider vinegar has also been found to help animals control their smell, heal skin conditions, and deter insects such as mosquitoes from animals.

MAKE YOUR DEODORANT

Odor on the body can be caused by some factors that range from sweet to bacteria, and it is most often strongest in areas of the body that are restricted by clothing or creased, allowing moisture to settle (such as the armpits) where bacteria can thrive. An alarming number of people are unaware that they're placing chemical-laden, store-bought deodorants directly onto a thin layer of skin that covers lymph nodes and veins in the armpit. This highway of blood-transporting veins and nodes absorbs the chemicals and additives in deodorants and antiperspirants and delivers them throughout the body in the blood stream. Because of the possibility of health hazards that can result from the chemicals used in these products, many consumers are opting for natural forms of deodorants that safely and more efficiently kill the cause of the odor without risking their health.

Apple cider vinegar can be used as an effective deodorant that does not pose health risks and boosts the body's overall health.

TO MAKE A HOMEMADE DEODORANT, COMBINE:

One tablespoon water • one tablespoon ACV

Apply the mixture to the armpit or area of odor with a cotton ball and allow to dry.

Not only does this application kill odor-causing and infection-breeding bacteria; it is absorbed into the blood stream and helps to assist the body's everyday functioning by ensuring the systems throughout the body receive necessary nutrients.

TO MAKE A PREVENTIVE DRINK, COMBINE:

1 cup water • one tablespoon ACV

Drink daily to reap the benefits of health-boosting vitamins, minerals, and antioxidants that prevent odor-causing bacteria from breeding within the body and on the skin's surface.

➢ WONDERS WITH WEIGHT LOSS

People have always looked for natural ways to reduce and manage their weight. Promoters of weight loss products are always introducing new products on a daily basis. It is important to note that the easier the weight loss solution, the higher the chances of success. One of the most overlooked natural products is the Apple Cider Vinegar weight loss solution. It has in recent times gained popularity due to research that has uncovered some of the benefits which were enjoyed long ago and had since been forgotten in modern times. Stop wasting money on expensive, ineffective and unnatural weight loss products and get back to the basics!

APPLE CIDER VINEGAR KEEPS PEOPLE FEELING SATIATED

A most acidic solution like vinegar has long been believed to help with weight loss among many people. Intake of apple cider vinegar is supposed to prolong the sensation of satiety thus making a person feel full for a long time.

Drinking apple cider vinegar before meals can help people immensely who want to lose weight. The reason why drinking apple cider vinegar gives the feeling of satiety is that it contains significant amounts of pectin. Apple cider vinegar contains the same amount of pectin as raw apples. It means that a glass of apple cider vinegar contains 1.5 grams of pectin as fresh apple thus the effects of eating an apple is just the same with drinking vinegar.

APPLE CIDER VINEGAR HELPS IMPROVE PROTEIN UTILIZATION

Another reason why apple cider vinegar can help with weight loss is that the acid helps with the digestion of proteins. Proteins serve as the basic unit or building blocks of different hormones and by increasing the amount of acid present in the stomach increases the ability of the availability of the stomach protein for hormone synthesis. Protein utilization can help the formation of hormones particularly growth hormones which keep the metabolism of the body active even if you are at rest or sleeping.

APPLE CIDER VINEGAR HELPS EFFECTIVELY BURN FATS IN THE STOMACH

Drinking apple cider vinegar can help stimulate the stomach, and a simulated stomach means efficient digestion. It also means that the fat is easily burned in the stomach. It is crucial that the stomach removes conditions that will cause diarrhea or constipation because they can be life threatening. Moreover, having food stored in the intestines for a long time means that unnecessary fats can be absorbed by the body thus causing higher visceral fats and triglycerides in the blood. With apple cider vinegar, it aids the stomach in effectively burning of fats as well as its excretion.

APPLE CIDER VINEGAR CAN IMPROVE UTILIZATION OF IRON

Iron is a key element that carries oxygen to the cells and holds them there. The intake of apple cider vinegar can help the release of iron in any food that you eat thus making it more available for the blood as well as for the muscle. Oxygen is essential for burning energy in the body as it serves as a starter in fuel. The ability of the apple cider vinegar to increase the utilization of iron as well as power consumption makes it very ideal for weight loss.

APPLE CIDER VINEGAR INCREASES YOUR INTEREST TO WHOLE FOODS

Intake of apple cider vinegar a few minutes before any meal can help increase your interest to eating whole foods. In fact, apple cider vinegar works at the beginning of the digestive process. When you take in apple cider vinegar, it stimulates your taste buds by producing more saliva. Once your taste buds are working well, it will easy for you to appreciate whole foods – foods that will help regulate your blood sugar level. It will help you prevent eating foods that are high in salt and fat.

APPLE CIDER VINEGAR CONTAINS POTASSIUM

Apples contain high amounts of potassium. When apple cider vinegar is taken regularly, it can help balance the sodium in your body. Sodium is an essential element that the body needs but too much of it can cause health problems like high blood pressure. Moreover, too much sodium also increases the amount of water weight that you can carry thus tempting you to eat more high-calorie food that can increase the risk of weight gain.

➢ APPETITE AND FAT LOSS

According to the 2006 Medscape Journal of Medicine, some of the benefits of Apple cider vinegar for weight loss include the fact that the vinegar has a role in blood sugar control and consequently leads to a suppressed appetite. Apple cider vinegar is also reported to prevent fat accumulation by influencing insulin production leading to weight loss. By stabilizing blood sugar, the apple cider vinegar helps control urges for carbohydrates and sugary foods as well as snacks which can also result in weight loss. This fact is supported by a 2004 study in diabetes care that confirmed vinegar to have fat burning properties too. It is also said that the vinegar from fresh apples contains pectin, a known soluble fiber that regulates cholesterol in the body.

Ever been on a diet, peering into your refrigerator, looking for something to stop your stomach from growling? Even though you've been able to stick to your diet, eat clean foods, and drink loads of water, you still find yourself hungry and with a seemingly insatiable appetite that is sure to lead to diet derailment in no time. Rather than give in to temptation or suffer through the feelings of starvation and deprivation, choose the healthy alternative: apple cider vinegar.

TO MAKE A DRINK, COMBINE:

2 cups water • one tablespoon ACV

To use, stir well, and sip throughout the day.

The enzymes and acetic acid in ACV normalize the acid levels (pH levels) of your stomach, reducing hunger pains and cravings, and resulting in decreased appetite. There are other theories about why ACV helps regulate appetite, too. One theory is that the acetic acid in ACV reduces the glycemic index of foods, which slows the rate that sugars are released into the blood stream, prolonging the feeling of satiety after a meal and reducing cravings. Another theory is that the pectin in ACV mixes with water/liquid and expands, leading to a decrease in appetite. Regardless of how it works, it does! The best part about this topic is that it's easy to make, and very portable making it a simple option to reach for instead of food you'd eat and regret later.

Place a sticky note or index card in your fridge or cabinet where your favorite craving foods are stored reminding you of your ACV appetite-suppressing option. This way, you see the reminder every time you reach for foods that aren't diet-friendly.

➤ DETOXIFICATION

FEWER TOXINS, LESS WEIGHT

Apple cider vinegar is said to work as a detoxification agent, and as we all know a body with fewer toxins has a more efficient metabolism which leads to greater weight loss. Being rich in acetic acid, apple cider vinegar slows the digestion of starches which reduces the rise in glucose that occurs after a meal. However, due to its highly acidic nature users are cautioned to take LESS than three tablespoons at a time. Alternatively, it should be diluted with water to reduce its acidity. It is also recommended that if you are on medication, you should consult your doctor to find out the possible reaction of the apple cider vinegar with your body and any drugs or supplements you currently take.

Apple cider vinegar also facilitates body detoxification as its natural acids usually bind toxins, eliminating them from the body. It helps in the breaking down of mucus throughout the body and aids in cleansing the lymphatic system allowing efficient lymphatic flow. It will translate to a greater removal of toxins from cells in the body. In cases of a sore throat, it has been found that apple cider vinegar can help in facilitating healing by clearing out the mucus and germs associated with the discomfort.

➤ DETOXIFY YOUR LIVER

Few people know what the liver does. The liver is an organ that secretes bile to aid in effective digestion, but its duties go far beyond that! The liver also protects and promotes one's vitality by:

- Filtering toxins and waste products in the blood
- Producing energy by manufacturing essential proteins and storing carbohydrates and other essential nutrients
- Properly metabolizing fats

Keeping the liver free of dangerous toxins that compromise its ability to function properly is a major step in maintaining overall health and wellness.

You can safeguard the optimal functioning of your liver by consuming a diet and living a lifestyle that presents the liver with a lighter workload:

- Eat a clean diet that includes whole foods like fruits, vegetables, nuts, and seeds
- Drink minimal alcohol
- Drink lots of clear fluids (preferably water)
- Avoid toxic substances like nicotine and drugs (prescription and otherwise)

Apple cider vinegar makes for the perfect partner in liver detoxification by contributing its variety of vitamins, minerals, and enzymes to maintain a healthy pH balance.

TO MAKE An LIVER-CLEANSING DRINK, COMBINE:

1 cup water • 1–2 teaspoons ACV • 1/2 teaspoon raw honey Drink three times a day.

Apple cider vinegar has long been used as an effective detoxification tool, and for a good reason! The primary goals of a detox are to:

- Cleanse the system of toxins, such as air and environmental pollutants, processed ingredients from foods, and chemicals from everyday products

- Assist the body's organ systems in ridding the body of built-up waste
- Replenish the body's stores of valuable vitamins and minerals essential for optimal functioning

An apple cider vinegar detox offers all of these benefits, and more, making it the perfect addition to a detoxification plan. It's simple, easy, and efficient, and sure to leave you feeling rejuvenated, refreshed, and healthfully replenished! A natural, organic option that offers a variety of vitamins, minerals, and essential nutrients, ACV can be the perfect supplement that provides cleansing properties and restorative vitamins and minerals, everything you need to ensure you're providing your body with what it needs during a detoxification program.

TO MAKE A SUPPLEMENTAL DETOX DRINK, COMBINE:

One tablespoon ACV • 2 cups water

Drink the ACV mixture in the morning, afternoon, and evening. If your rehab includes meals, drink the mixture 30 minutes before meals.

A typical detoxification plan lasts for one to seven days and sometimes includes whole foods. Usually, you start by consuming only liquids; then you might slowly introduce whole foods. While most people opt to use a liquid-only cleanse to allow the body to rid itself of waste and start "fresh" after the detox is completed, there is a significant benefit to including certain whole foods: Adding fiber will assist the body's digestive system in purging waste.

A detox plan that includes ACV provides so many advantages:

- Beneficial enzymes and acetic acid that help neutralize stomach acids
- Added fiber, which forms a gel in the gut and helps to remove toxins and waste
- Helps the liver and other organs that play essential roles in detoxifying the body remove toxins while replenishing stores of vitamins and minerals needed to operate more efficiently
- Powerful antioxidants that boost the immune system and safeguard one's health throughout the detoxification process
- Many people who consume ACV have reported an increase in energy levels.

➤ CURES AND REMEDIES

Apple cider vinegar is used for many natural treatments and cures. It has been considered to be one of the only all—inclusive home remedies that treat a numerous amount of ailments and conditions. Apple cider vinegar is also a highly versatile ingredient that can easily be found in many different forms at your local grocery store. All the cures that apple cider vinegar claims to offer are incredibly useful. However, you need to make sure to use only the purest apple cider vinegar for it to have an effect. Raw, unpasteurized and homemade vinegar is the best and most effective.

ACHES, PAINS & BITES

Drinking two teaspoons of ACV has been shown to help ease leg aches, menstrual cramps, hot flashes and even night sweats. It also stops the pain of any insect burns, bites, and stings due to its containing of many antibacterial properties. The discomfort of sunburns and varicose veins could easily be soothed by the applying of lightly diluted apple cider vinegar because of the natural antibacterial and anti-fungal properties it offers.

SOOTHE STOMACHACHES

Stomachaches can be caused by some disruptions that range from psychological stresses and poor lifestyle choices to bad habits and prolonged exposure to unhealthy irritants. You might experience acute stomach aches once in a while, or you might be plagued with less extreme but longer-lasting versions. No matter why you get stomachaches, you can effectively minimize their severity, frequency, and duration by attacking the root of the problem, rather than treating the symptoms that result.

Ensuring that your digestive system, from your saliva to your colon, is running efficiently, you can prevent stomachaches from occurring, and treat them once they strike. By regulating the pH balance of your entire digestive system, ACV begins fighting the causes of illnesses. By fighting off bacteria, viruses, and possible irritants that could further exacerbate an illness, ACV can aid in relieving the body of possible diseases or invaders that can cause or increase uneasiness.

TO MAKE A DRINK, COMBINE:

1 cup water • one tablespoon ACV

Sip the solution over a period of 30 minutes to experience relief from stomach aches

EASE A SORE THROAT

A sore throat can come on unexpectedly and can be an isolated experience or a symptom of a far more severe condition. Pharyngitis, which means "inflammation of the throat," is the medical term for a sore throat. While it has some causes that range from infection to irritation, a sore throat should be treated as soon as the scratchiness, irritation, and pain arise. Whether the crux of the issue is viral or bacterial, apple cider vinegar is a natural remedy that provides nutritional benefits that calm from the inside out. Containing some naturally occurring vitamins, minerals, enzymes, and antioxidants—along with antiviral and antibiotic properties—that work together in soothing a sore throat, ACV in its natural, unfiltered, organic state can perform the job of some medications all on its own!

TO MAKE A DRINK, COMBINE:

1 cup warmed water • one tablespoon ACV • 1 teaspoon honey (if creating a tonic to drink)

Gargle the mixture by 1/4-cup gulps, or drink the tonic heated with the added teaspoon of honey to kill germs in the mouth and throat as you swallow the mixture.

The vitamin C contained in ACV also provides immunity-boosting effects by fending off illness while also strengthening the immune system.

SOOTHE SINUSITIS

Sinusitis, also known as a sinus infection, is a condition caused by a microorganism (in the form of a bacteria, virus, or fungus) that grows within the air pockets of the sinus and causes a blockage. While some experience sinusitis once in a while, many sufferers find they have chronic sinus problems. As a result of the infection, the sinuses swell and begin producing an abnormal amount of mucus. As the infection persists, the inflammation and mucus cause the traditional sinusitis symptoms of headaches, facial tenderness, sinus pressure and pain, fever, dark and cloudy nasal discharge, stuffiness, sore throat, cough, and even toothaches. While many cases of sinusitis require antibiotics, some sinusitis sufferers can find relief long before the infection has grown to the point of requiring prescription medications. Over-the-counter relievers are effective in soothing sore throats, relieving pain and fevers, and drying up mucus, but they can also deliver undesirable side effects. For sinusitis sufferers choosing to use natural remedies before turning to more extreme measures, apple cider vinegar is the perfect option.

Containing antibacterial and antiviral properties, apple cider vinegar is packed with essential antioxidants, vitamins, and minerals that combine to combat infections and soothe symptoms. Reinforcing the body's immune system with loads of natural vitamin C, ACV provides support to a sinusitis sufferer by alleviating the symptoms, pinpointing the cause of the condition, and repairing the immune system.

TO MAKE A SOOTHING DRINK TO COMBAT THE SOURCE OF SINUSITIS (BACTERIAL, VIRAL, OR OTHERWISE), COMBINE:

1 tablespoon ACV • 1 cup hot water

Drink three times daily.

TO MAKE A STEAM TREATMENT, COMBINE IN A POT:

1 cup ACV • 4 cups water

Inhale the vapors as the steam is produced.

RELIEVE LEG CRAMPS

Cramps in the muscles throughout the body can be caused by issues such as:

- Nutrient deficiencies
- Dehydration
- Excessive wear and tear resulting from exercise or bouts of physical endurance
- Poor circulation

Whether the leg cramps you experience result from one of these possible causes or seem to have been brought on by another factor, your local pharmacy probably boasts a vast array of anti-inflammatory pills, tonics, and topical creams that promise to provide relief. While many of these solutions may be effective, they may provide only a temporary relief and often come with a host of possible undesirable side effects. If you find yourself suffering from leg cramps, try these ACV options.

TO MAKE A QUICK-ACTING TONIC, COMBINE:

One tablespoon ACV • 2 cups water

Drink 1–3 times daily until symptoms subside.

TO MAKE A SOOTHING BATH SOLVENT, COMBINE:

Tub full of warm water • 1 cup ACV

Soak in the mixture for up to 30 minutes to relieve lactic acid buildup, stimulate circulation, and remove toxins.

The organic, unfiltered variety can replenish the body's stores of valuable vitamins and minerals that are depleted when cramping and muscle soreness occur.

TO MAKE A TOPICAL SOLUTION, DAMPEN A WET TOWEL WITH ACV.

Apply the towel directly to the cramping area of the leg to relieve lactic acid buildup, stimulate circulation, and remove toxins.

Apple cider vinegar contains some reparative vitamins and minerals that have been shown to provide pain relief in muscles and joints. Said to improve circulation of the blood, ACV has long been used to alleviate muscle cramping and soreness by stimulating blood flow throughout the body and delivering higher volumes of oxygenated blood to the areas in need.

RELIEVE MUSCLE STIFFNESS

Lactic acid is the normal byproduct produced by muscles following the processing of essential proteins. The buildup of lactic acid in the muscles is what can cause stiffness and pain in areas such as the neck, back, butt, legs, and arms. While stretching is the most efficient way to cure muscle stiffness—because it allows the muscles to release the lactic acid into the blood to be carried away as waste—many muscle stiffness sufferers opt for over-the-counter treatments. Unfortunately, most relieve the pain only temporarily, and in some cases even aggravate the condition! Luckily, lactic acid buildup in the muscles can be naturally treated by stretching of the stiff areas and using various apple cider vinegar applications. ACV contains acetic acid and vitamins and minerals that aid in the processing of elements such as lactic acid.

TO MAKE A DRINK, COMBINE:

1 cup water • two teaspoons ACV

TO MAKE A SOOTHING BATH, COMBINE:

Tub full of water • 2 cups ACV

Soaking for up to 30 minutes allows the nutrients, acids, and enzymes in ACV to pull toxins from the body, enabling the body to more efficiently rid the muscles and blood of lactic acid buildup.

TO MAKE A TOPICAL TREATMENT, COMBINE IN A BOWL:

1 cup water • 1/4 cup ACV

Warm the mixture, then submerge a towel in the solution, ring out the excess, and place the sheet directly on the site of stiffness for 15 minutes at a time.

LESSEN JOINT PAIN

Pain experienced in the joints can be due to a buildup of toxins within the joint cavity or surrounding muscle and connective tissues. Because it is the toxicity in joints that can result in uncomfortable irritation and inflammation, many over-the-counter medications can be helpful in alleviating symptoms but may do so only temporarily, treating the symptoms but not the source of the issue. Plus, they can contain harmful chemicals and additives. By addressing the cause of the joint pain with ACV instead, you can alleviate the symptoms and prevent the symptoms' return efficiently and naturally.

As a pain-relieving alternative to over-the-counter medications, apple cider vinegar provides healing properties that promote the optimal functioning of some systems, boosting the body's overall immunity while also focusing on reducing the toxicity of the joints where the pain is being experienced. The naturally occurring enzymes and antioxidants within apple cider vinegar act to combat the build-up of the body's waste products that can accumulate in joints and surrounding tissues. These enzymes and antioxidants bind with the toxic substances and flush them out in the blood stream and digestive systems. You can find the aloe vera juice used in this tonic at health food stores and some grocery stores.

TO MAKE A DRINK, COMBINE:

1 cup water • two tablespoons organic aloe vera juice • one tablespoon ACV

Drink daily.

TO MAKE AN ON-THE-SPOT TREATMENT, SOAK A WET TOWEL WITH ACV.

Apply to the site of joint pain, allowing the ACV to help draw out toxins from the area. Leave application at the location of joint pain for over an hour. Repeat as needed.

TO MAKE A SOOTHING SOAK, COMBINE:

Tub full of warm water • 4 cups ACV

Soak for 30–60 minutes to allow the properties of ACV to draw toxins out of the body naturally, minimizing the pain in the affected areas.

ALLEVIATE HEADACHES

Resulting from dehydration, stress, sinus pressure, muscle tension, elements of a poor diet, or more dangerous conditions, headaches can be a terrible experience that ranges from merely frustrating to frequent and debilitating. Many over-the-counter medications and heavy-duty prescriptions are recommended for the treatment of headaches, but these can contain some unhealthy elements that could produce undesirable side effects.

Apple cider vinegar is one of the most beneficial natural treatments for a problem because of the vast amount of vitamins, minerals, acids, and enzymes it contains. Delivering essential nutrients to the body is a major step in migraine treatment and prevention because it ensures that the body's systems have adequate fuel to perform optimally. ACV also helps headaches by:

- Eliminating possible physical causes of headaches such as dehydration
- Improving blood quality by removing toxins
- Improving circulation by boosting metabolic functioning
- Easing muscle tension

TO MAKE An HEADACHE-REDUCING DRINK, COMBINE:

1 cup decaffeinated tea • one tablespoon ACV

Drink every hour until a headache dissipates.

REDUCE SWELLING

While most instances of swelling occur as a result of injuries or trauma, it can also arise from a poor diet or displaced pressure. However, the swelling started, as long as serious injuries like fractures and tendon or ligament damage are ruled out, you can actually alleviate swelling safely and in the comfort of your own home with apple cider vinegar treatments!

Apple cider vinegar can be used to treat swelling by:

- Contributing essential vitamins, minerals, enzymes, and acids to detoxifying the body
- Replenishing important stores of nutrients
- Improving circulation and blood flow to the affected area
- Repairing damaged tissues

TO MAKE A DRINK, COMBINE:

1 cup water • two tablespoons aloe vera juice • one tablespoon ACV

Drink daily to reduce swelling and prevent further injury caused by inflammation.

TO MAKE A SOAK THAT CAN RELIEVE SWELLING BY DRAWING TOXINS OUT OF THE BODY, IMPROVE CIRCULATION, AND ASSIST IN NUTRIENT DELIVERY TO THE AFFECTED AREA, COMBINE:

Tub full of warm water • 2–4 cups ACV

Soak for 30–45 minutes, allowing the ACV mixture to penetrate the affected area and treat it from the inside out.

TO MAKE A SPOT TREATMENT, SOAK A WASHCLOTH WITH:

1 cup ACV • 1/2 cup water

Sit with the swollen area elevated, and drape the washcloth over the affected area for 30 minutes at a time every hour until the swelling subsides.

RELIEVE EARACHES

With powerful antibacterial, antiviral, and antiseptic properties, apple cider vinegar can be used as an active agent in getting rid of ear pain. Delivering powerful nutrients that also contribute to the healing process by killing the infection, reducing inflammation, and minimizing the pain that results, ACV can be an effective preventive measure as well.

TO MAKE EARDROPS, COMBINE:

1/4 cup ACV • 1/8 cup water

Warm the solution to body temperature. Drop the solution into your ear for 10 minutes at a time, allow to seep out slowly, and repeat every hour as needed. This process can be repeated multiple times per day, as necessary, to reduce pain resulting from the infection.

TO MAKE A DRINK THAT CAN BE USED FOR PAIN RELIEF OR AS A PREVENTIVE MEASURE, COMBINE:

1 cup water • one tablespoon ACV

For pain relief, drink three times daily until an earache is gone

Drink once daily after the infection has cleared as a preventive measure.

An earache is an uncomfortable condition that can be caused by bacterial or viral infections of the ear canal or any of the outlying areas. By acting swiftly to kill infections that could be causing the earache, you can minimize the painful symptoms that result as well as the duration of an earache. To restore health to the ear's affected area, many pain sufferers turn to over-the-counter medications that can contain harmful chemicals and additives. Not only can this cause damage to the ear or further aggravate the condition; it is important to keep in mind that the ear and its canals to the inner workings of the body are delicate, making some wary of using chemically created products for relief.

EASE BACKACHES

Backaches can affect every aspect of your daily life. Sitting, standing, walking, driving, and performing the simplest of tasks can become painful activities when you're suffering from a backache. Whether the cause is in the muscles, tissues, bones, or nerves, apple cider vinegar can provide you with the relief you need. Rich in minerals and vitamins that can deliver numerous benefits to multiple systems of the body, ACV has long been used to fight inflammation, which is the most common cause of backaches. ACV provides specific relief to backache sufferers by supplying ample amounts of those essential nutrients needed to repair and restore health to the systems most affected during backaches. Forgo the over-the-counter, chemical-laden medications that promise relief, and opt for this natural alternative that not only calms the site of inflammation but also works to optimize the functioning of the systems affected.

Lactic acid buildup in muscles, calcium issues within the bones, and potassium deficiencies in the nervous system are just a few possible causes of backaches that can all be assisted with the nutrients provided by ACV. The calcium, magnesium, and silica in ACV:

- Fight inflammation
- Boost the body's immune system functioning
- Improve blood flow and blood quality
- Assist in pain relief by reducing inflammation

Following are several ways to use ACV to help you deal with backaches.

TO MAKE A DAILY TONIC, COMBINE:

1 cup water • 1 tablespoon ACV

Drink daily.

TO MAKE A TOPICAL RELIEF, COMBINE:

Tub full of warm water • 2–4 cups ACV

Soak for 30–60 minutes at a time.

Providing relief and preventive treatment, ACV has helped countless backache sufferers return to their pain-free daily lives!

RELIEVE BURNS

Surprisingly, apple cider vinegar has long been used as a first-aid treatment for minor burns. Because of its acidity, most people are surprised at the suggestion of using ACV as an injury treatment, assuming the acids would aggravate the injury or cause additional pain. Quite the contrary, apple cider vinegar has potent properties that assist in relieving the pain of an injury, soothing the site of irritation, and delivering nutrients that help the healing process while also safeguarding the injury suffered from an infection. The naturally occurring enzymes, acids, and vitamins and minerals of ACV synergistically help to:

- Reduce inflammation
- Speed the healing process
- Prevent germs, bacteria, and viruses from entering the body through the wound
- Promote reparative skin cell production

Whether your burn is the result of hot liquids or chemicals coming into contact with your skin, first treat the affected area with a cool compress or a cool soak to return the affected area's temperature to normal. Then, proceed with an ACV soak.

<u>TO MAKE AN ACV SOAK, COMBINE:</u>

2 cups water • 1/2 cup ACV

Submerge the affected area for 15 minutes at a time over the course of 2–3 hours.

This combination has shown to be an effective method of treatment that can be used for days following the burn, helping to soothe a burn site and jump-start the healing process. Following the soaking treatments, you can also utilize the many components of ACV to reduce the pain and inflammation at the location of the burn.

TO MAKE A BANDAGE AID, COMBINE:

2 cups water • 1/2 cup ACV

Soak the gauze in the ACV mixture and wrap the wound loosely. This process continues the delivery of healing components to the site of the burn.

HEAL BRUISES

A bruise is the visible result of subcutaneous blood vessels being broken, and it can be accompanied with sensitivity or pain in the affected area. Because few topical treatments are suggested for treating bruises, most people adopt a "wait it out" mentality and allow the injury to heal on its own. However, there are ways to speed the healing process of an injury and reduce the unsightly appearance of the red, purple, green, or black in the area. One such method is a double dose of apple cider vinegar that can be taken orally and also applied to the site of the bruise, helping to speed the healing process and reduce the inflammation and discoloration that results.

ACV helps bruises by:

- Delivering acids and enzymes that assist the blood in its cleansing process and help the body to detoxify the blood of waste products such as the broken blood vessels
- Supplying vitamin C and beta carotene to support the immune system's functioning, fight infection that could result from the trauma that caused the bruise, and help to repair and regenerate valuable blood cells

TO MAKE A HEALING DRINK, COMBINE:

1 cup water • one tablespoon ACV

Drink once daily as symptoms persist.

TO MAKE A TOPICAL TREATMENT FOR BRUISES, COMBINE:

1/4 cup water • 1/4 cup ACV

Soak a washcloth in the mixture and apply directly to the site of the injury, helping to improve blood flow and circulation and assisting in the healing process.

RELIEVE INSECT BITES

Being bitten or stung by an insect can set off a series of reactions that can range from mildly uncomfortable to life-threatening. While most insect stings and bites are not fatal, they can create skin conditions that itch, burn, or sting, and can last for hours, days, or even weeks! Use apple cider vinegar as a healing treatment for bites you have—and even to avoid future bites!

The naturally occurring acids and enzymes in apple cider vinegar act as a deterrent against bugs that can bite and sting. Able to detect the distasteful and aromatic elements of ACV from afar, bugs are discouraged from even approaching an individual that has ACV on the skin.

TO MAKE A BUG SPRAY, COMBINE IN A SPRAY BOTTLE:

1 cup ACV • 1/4 cup water

Sprinkle the skin with the mixture or use a towel to apply the solution to the skin and actually deter bugs from stinging or biting.

To make a topical treatment for soothing stings and bites, apply undiluted ACV to the skin with a towel or cotton ball every 15 minutes. Not only does this prevent inflammation at the site of the sting or bite; it also helps to neutralize the venom excreted by the insect.

Do not hesitate to seek immediate medical attention if you think your particular reaction warrants medical intervention.

➤ ACNE

The Lactic and malic acids found inside of apple cider vinegar have been proven to soften and exfoliate the skin, reducing red marks on the face. Apple cider vinegar was even shown to help tone skin and creates the proper pH balance resulting in the reduction of acne. Apple cider vinegar is a highly efficient, incredibly low-cost skin care product for acne. Remember, apple cider vinegar is very acidic, and if you have the fair or sensitive skin, you should always be sure to dilute the solution with water to avoid unnecessary irritation significantly.

Acne sufferers have long searched for the resolution of blemishes that can appear on the face, neck, chest, back, and arms. Prescription medications and over-the-counter treatments are sometimes expensive, ineffective, or loaded with harsh chemicals and additives. To treat the condition safely, naturally, and actually, acne sufferers can use apple cider vinegar in some ways.

Apple cider vinegar can be used in four effective treatment options (as a soak, tonic, topical treatment, or facial mask) that are inexpensive, easy to use, and completely risk-free!

The procedures that include apple cider vinegar, when applied directly to the skin in a soak/bath, facial cleanser, or mask, are intended to achieve some regulatory and restorative balances in the skin that will help to alleviate the causes of acne and prevent future occurrences. When applied directly to the skin, apple cider vinegar's antioxidants, vitamins, minerals, acids, and enzymes work synergistically to:

- Restore an average pH to the skin
- Regulate oil production that can lead to the clogging of pores
- Reduce inflammation at the site of blemishes
- Improve circulation in the skin to lessen the appearance of blemishes and redness that so often accompany acne

TO MAKE A SOAK, COMBINE:

Tub full of water • 2–4 cups ACV

Soak for up to 30 minutes.

TO MAKE A TONIC, COMBINE:

1 cup water • one tablespoon ACV

Drink daily.

TO MAKE A TOPICAL TREATMENT, COMBINE:

1/4 cup ACV • 1/8 cup water

Apply to skin as needed.

TO MAKE A FACIAL MASK, COMBINE:

1/2 mashed avocado • 1/4 cup ACV

Apply evenly to face, allowing to sit for 10 minutes daily.

➤ EASE INDIGESTION

While many people use the terms "heartburn" and "indigestion" interchangeably, they are two different conditions. Heartburn is defined as discomfort in the stomach associated with digesting food. Heartburn can be caused by some factors acting individually or combined, and it strikes people of both genders, all ages, and, surprisingly, even those who adhere to the strictest of healthy diets. Here are some common causes:

- Overeating
- Eating spicy or acidic foods
- Allergic reactions or intolerances to specific foods such as gluten, lactose, or excessively fatty or greasy foods

The underlying problem that leads to all cases of indigestion is inadequate stomach acid for digestion. Antacids are the common prescription for indigestion, yet they rarely cure it because they don't address the problem. By calming the stomach's acidic state naturally with a balancing acid (not an antacid), the stomach returns to a healthy pH balance.

When consuming ACV, you supplement the inadequate stomach acid with a less intense version—acetic acid. Safely, easily, and naturally, the acetic acid can help soothe the symptoms of indigestion.

TO MAKE A DRINK, COMBINE:

1 cup water • 2–4 teaspoons ACV

To use, sip the concoction over a period of 20–30 minutes. You should feel the relief of the indigestion symptoms. Again, sip over a period of 20–30 minutes.

➢ AVOID BACTERIAL CYSTITIS

Bacterial cystitis is a medical term that is used interchangeably with the better-known term "urinary tract infection" or UTI. Cystitis is defined as an inflammation of the bladder, most commonly caused by bacteria. The alternative to the bacterial cause is interstitial cystitis. The bacterial version of cystitis more often occurs in women, but it can also be experienced by men and children; women are especially susceptible to the condition because of their shorter urethras, which are more easily exposed to harmful bacteria. The situation starts out feeling like a tingling sensation and can then become severe, with symptoms that cause the sufferer to feel the frequent urge to urinate, with or without urine being expelled, and can include pain and burning sensations experienced during urination. Because bacterial cystitis is a bacterial infection of the bladder, antibiotics are the proper course of treatment, but natural methods can be used to prevent and alleviate the condition.

Packed with valuable vitamins and minerals that assist in flushing the body of toxins such as the harmful bacteria that contribute to this uncomfortable condition, apple cider vinegar makes for the perfect preventive option in stopping bacterial cystitis before it starts. There are two ways to do this:

<u>TO MAKE A DRINK, COMBINE:</u>

1 cup water • one tablespoon ACV

Drink daily. Many women reports experiencing fewer incidences of bacterial cystitis than before starting an ACV regimen, and they experienced a reduced severity of symptoms when they consumed the concoction following the onset of the condition.

You can also try this bathing method:

COMBINE IN A BATHTUB:

1 cup ACV • Tub full of warm water

Soak for 30 minutes. This bath alleviates symptoms by killing bacteria in the urethra.

➢ SPEED UP METABOLISM

A fast metabolism is something that only "skinny" people have, right? Wrong! Genetics do play a significant role in metabolism, but any person can improve his or her rate of metabolism naturally. Try this invigorating ACV recipe:

TO MAKE A DRINK, COMBINE:

1 cup green tea • two tablespoons ACV • 1 tablespoon lemon juice • one teaspoon ground cayenne pepper

To use, drink this metabolism-boosting tonic 30 minutes before every meal.

The combination of caffeinated green tea, internal-temperature-raising cayenne pepper, and multiple vitamins and minerals in lemon juice and ACV promotes proper metabolic functioning, improves fat burning, and increases energy levels.

Along with this drink, try these simple lifestyle changes to boost your metabolic rates in a matter of weeks:

- Implement a strength-training routine designed to increase fat-burning muscle mass
- Eat smaller meals more frequently throughout the day
- Incorporate 30-minute bouts of cardiovascular exercise 4–6 days per week

➢ ACID REFLUX

If acid reflux is the result of an imbalance of stomach acids, then drinking a single tablespoon of apple cider vinegar can significantly help to relax and ease that discomfort. Apple cider vinegar was proven to help as it was one of the oldest prescribed medicinal practices for acidic problems and improper digestion. Many experts have even stated that apple cider vinegar is the best natural remedy to relieve your acid reflux and indigestion - almost immediately.

➢ REDUCE FLATULENCE

There are few things as embarrassing as excessive flatulence. Embarrassing, uncomfortable, and difficult to deal with, excessive gas and flatulence is a condition for which over-the-counter remedies run in the thousands. Chemically manufactured pills and drinks that promise to reduce the incidence of gas may be active, but they often include many chemicals and ingredients you can't pronounce.

While multiple medical conditions can cause excessive gas, most people who experience sporadic bouts of bloating and gas can point to unhealthy foods as the cause. Unhealthy diets wreak havoc on the digestive system, leaving excessive gas in their wake. However, even those who eat clean foods full of fibrous roughage, such as cruciferous vegetables (broccoli, cauliflower, etc.), can suffer from excessive gas buildup and frequent flatulence.

No matter what causes gas, ACV can help alleviate it. By combining a diet of healthy whole foods that calm gas-producing conditions such as honey, fennel, ginger, flax, cinnamon, and pineapple with all-natural ACV tonics that treat gas, you can experience far less flatulence. The volatile acids and enzymes of ACV help to alleviate gas production and flatulence by negating the gas-producing elements and processes involved.

TO MAKE A TONIC TO TREAT GAS, COMBINE:

1 cup water • one teaspoon honey • one teaspoon peppermint extract • 1/2 teaspoon cinnamon • one tablespoon ACV.

Drink daily.

Chapter 5: Health Risks Associated with Apple Cider Vinegar Diet

All diet regimens have drawbacks, and this includes the apple cider vinegar diet. Even if apple cider vinegar diet is easy to follow and it has a lot of benefits aside from weight loss, it comes with several drawbacks that you need to be aware of. Since apple cider vinegar requires you to take a certain amount of acetic acid each day, this will significantly affect your health in the long run. In the study conducted by Karl Lhotta (et. al) in 1998 entitled Hypokalemia, Hyperreninemia, and Osteoporosis in a Patient Ingesting Large Amounts of Cider Vinegar, it noted that high dosage of apple cider vinegar could induce the following reactions to the body:

Consumption of large doses of apple cider vinegar can lower the potassium levels in the body which can affect the bone density leading to osteoporosis.

In theory, excessive use of apple cider vinegar can cause hypokalemia and hyperreninemia which are conditions that relate to having low potassium in the blood. In most cases, people who suffer from these diseases show symptoms like high blood pressure and cardiac arrests.

Apple cider vinegar also contains chromium which can alter insulin levels. Prolonged usage of apple cider vinegar can also pose problems to those who have diabetes. Intake should be controlled, or dieters who are planning to take on the apple cider vinegar diet should consult their doctors for such possible side effects.

Since apple cider vinegar contains acetic acid, consumption of pure apple cider vinegar can cause esophageal burns is especially true if you are taking apple cider vinegar pills which tend to be caught in the throat.

There are health risks that are involved in taking in apple cider vinegar, and it is important that you consider these risks to understand whether this particular diet regimen is right for you or not.

Chapter 6: Cooking with Apple Cider

HEALTHY DRINKS

1. APPLE CIDER VINEGAR DRINK

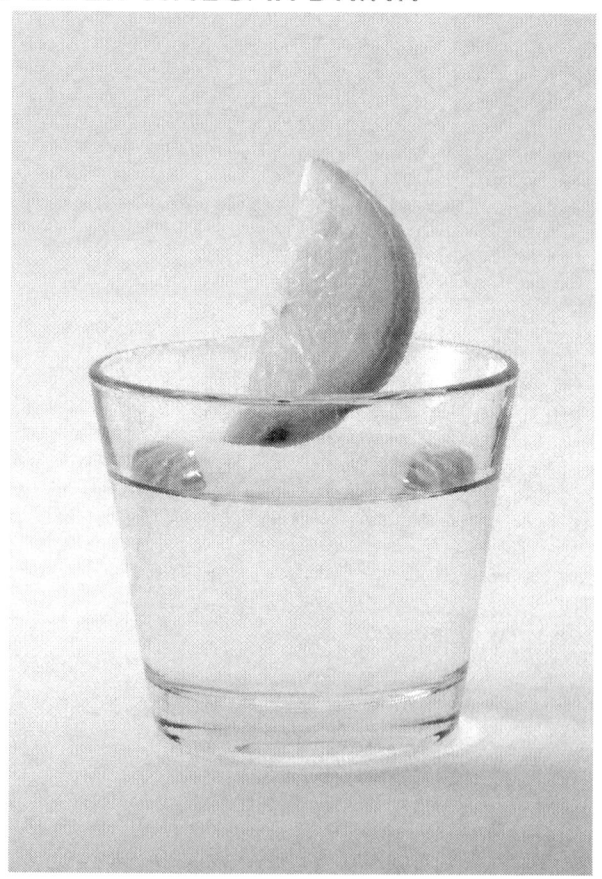

Nutritional Information per 1 Serving:
 Energy (calories): 21 kcal
 Protein: 0.05 g
 Fat: 0.06 g
 Carbohydrates: 5.25 g
 Gluten-free
 Vegan

Ingredients (1 serving):
- 1 to 3 Tbsp. Apple Cider Vinegar
- 8 oz. cold water

Optional:
- 1 tsp. Honey or Stevia to taste
- Fresh ginger root (juice or grind)
- Fresh lemon juice to taste (Lemon juice pH is more acidic than ACV)

Directions:

1. Mix the ingredients in a glass jar. You can also to shake it for a minute until frothy. Generally, drink this on an empty stomach, but some people get an irritated stomach for a short time afterward.
2. Should that happen to you, try drinking an extra glass of water first. Recipes have varied from 1 teaspoon to 3 Tablespoon.
3. The original recipes call for honey because honey adds enzymes and vitamins that aid digestion.

2. ALMOND LATTE

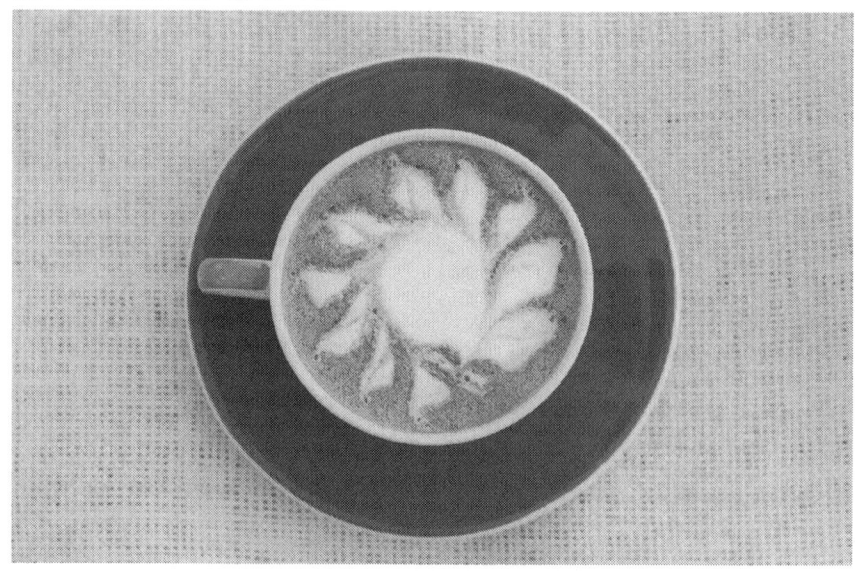

Nutritional Information per 1 Serving:
Energy (calories): 122 kcal
Protein: 1.95 g
Fat: 3 g
Carbohydrates: 22.51 g
Gluten-free
Vegan

Ingredients (1 serving):

- 1 cup hot green tea, double strength
- 1 cup almond milk
- 1 Tbsp. Apple Cider Vinegar
- Sugar, Stevia or Honey to taste

Directions:

1. Mix the ingredients
2. Enjoy the taste throughout the day.

3. GREEN TEA GINGER HOT TONIC

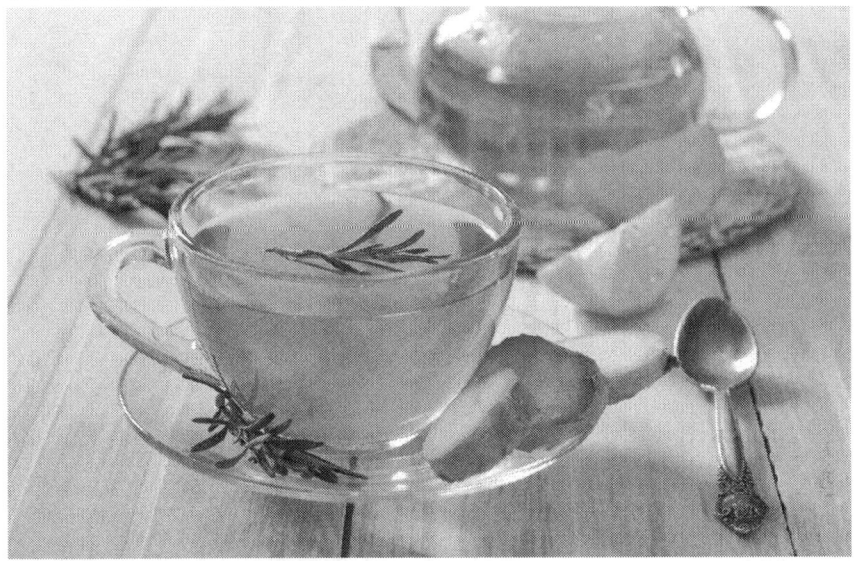

Nutritional Information per 1 Serving:

Energy (calories): 7 kcal
Protein: 0.04 g
Fat: 0.02 g
Carbohydrates: 2.2 g
Gluten-free
Vegan

Ingredients (1 serving):
- Steep green tea with chopped, thin slices of peeled fresh ginger.
- 1 Tbsp. Apple Cider Vinegar
- Sugar, Stevia or Honey to taste

Directions:
1. Mix the ingredients
2. Drink green tea, hot or cold, freshly made throughout the day

4. REFRESHING APPLE LEMON GINGER DRINK

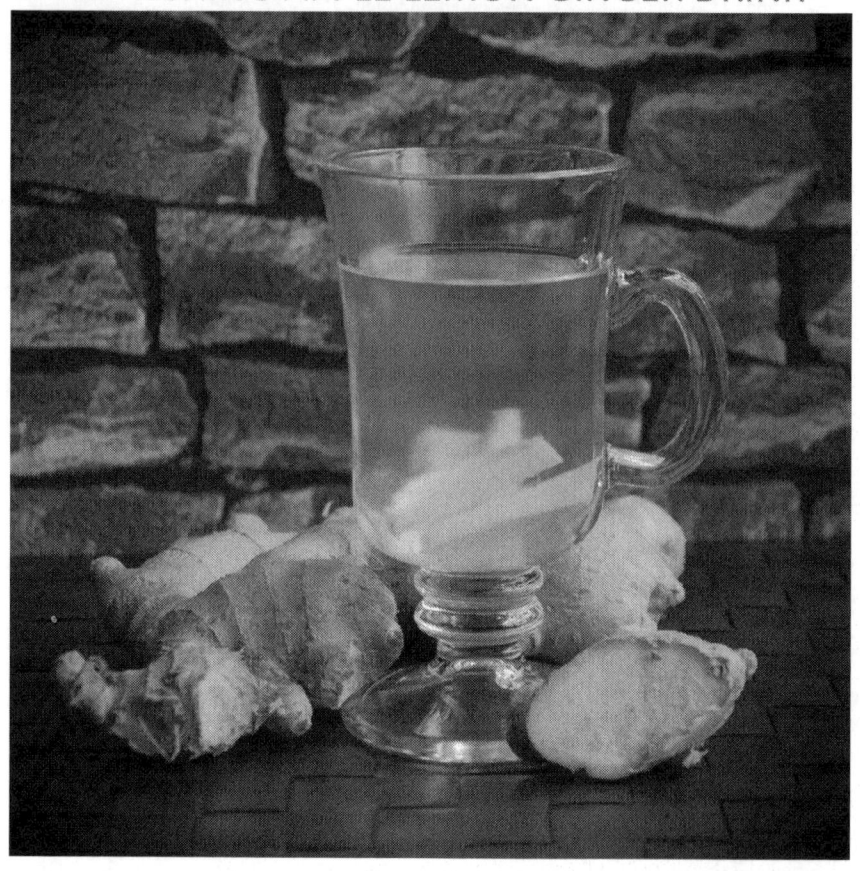

Nutritional Information per 1 Serving:
　Energy (calories): 210 kcal
　Protein: 1.13 g
　Fat: 0.74 g
　Carbohydrates: 54.17 g
　Gluten-free
　Vegan

Ingredients (2 servings):

- 2 Apples
- 1 Lemon
- Ginger to taste
- 2 cups Water
- 3 Tbsp. ACV
- Sugar, Stevia or Honey to taste

Directions:
1. Juice the apples, lemon, and ginger.
2. Add the ACV. If blending, Add water.
3. This recipe can be made as a hot or cold drink.
4. Adding 1 tsp. cinnamon will also make it tasty.

APPLE CIDER VINEGAR DRESSING AND SAUCES

5. CLASSIC APPLE CIDER VINEGAR DRESSING

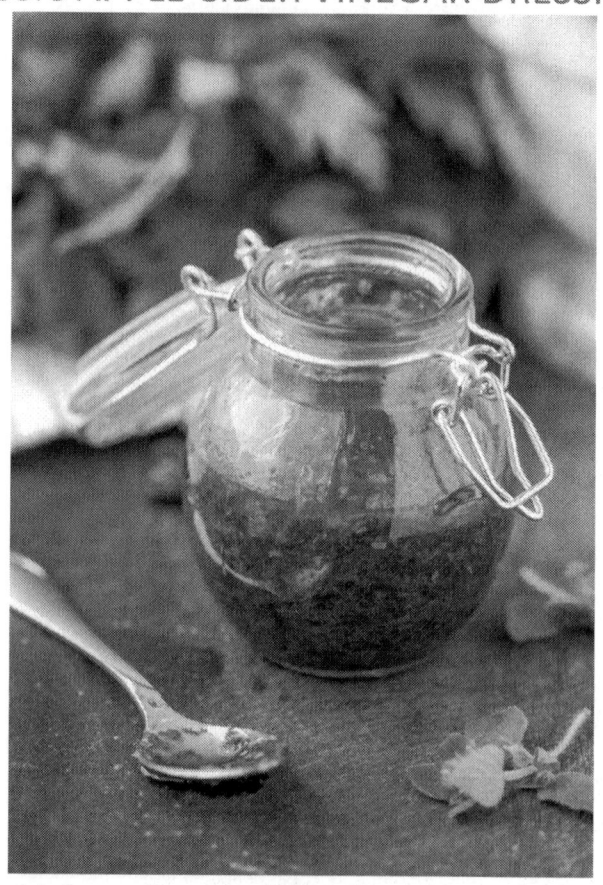

Nutritional Information per 1 Serving:
    Energy (calories): 47 kcal
    Protein: 0.55 g
    Fat: 0.22 g
    Carbohydrates: 11.02 g
    Gluten-free
    Vegan

Ingredients (1 serving):

- 2 Tbs. Apple Cider Vinegar
- Juice of 1 Fresh Large Lemon
- 1/2 cup Celery, strung, 1/8" chop
- 1 tsp. Honey or Stevia to taste
- 1/2 tsp. Rubbed Rosemary or Fresh Basil

Options:

- Add Water to thin as needed
- 2 tsp. Whole Grain mustard (no sugar)

Directions:

1. Add the ingredients into a glass jar. Shake for one minute.
2. Serve over greens and salad vegetables.
3. Go to top

6. LOVELY APPLE SAUCE

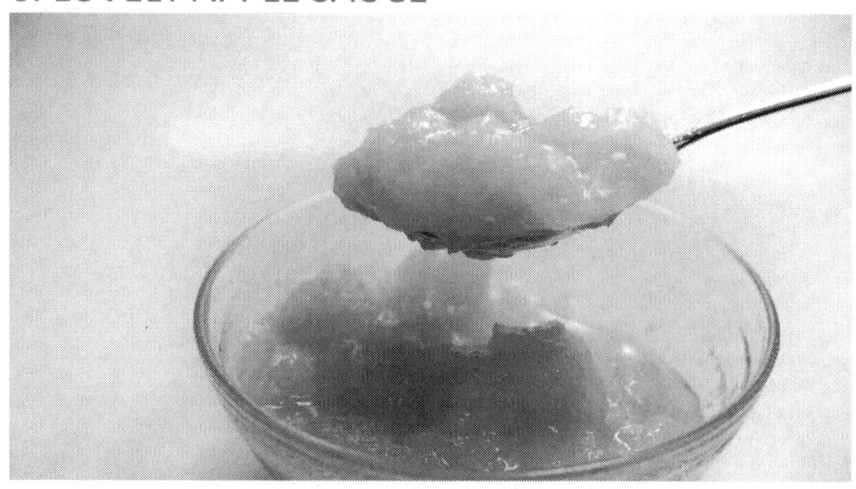

Nutritional Information per 1 Serving:
  Energy (calories): 100 kcal
  Protein: 0.48 g
  Fat: 0.32 g
  Carbohydrates: 26.45 g
  Gluten-free
  Vegan

Ingredients (4 servings):

- 1 Package of pre-sliced apples (3-4 apples)
- 3 Tbs. of Apple Cider Vinegar

Directions:

1. Put into a puree and blend
2. Great for fruit salads.

7. EXQUISITE CREAMY POPPY SEED DRESSING

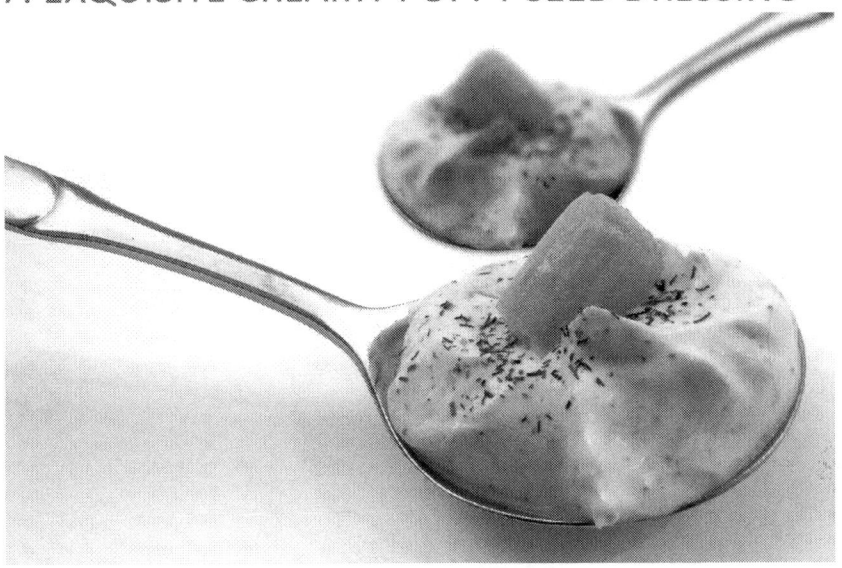

Nutritional Information per 1 Serving:
  Energy (calories): 129 kcal
  Protein: 12.44 g
  Fat: 2.29 g
  Carbohydrates: 15.75 g
  Gluten-free

Ingredients (2 servings):

- 1 Tbs. of poppy seeds
- 1 Tbs. of honey
- 8 oz. of Greek yogurt, plain
- 1 Tbs. of apple cider vinegar
- 1 Tbs. of orange juice
- salt
- pepper

Directions:

1. Mix all ingredients.
2. Season according to your taste.
3. Leave in the refrigerator.

SALADS

8. APPETIZING POTATO SALAD WITH CORNICHONS AND RADISHES

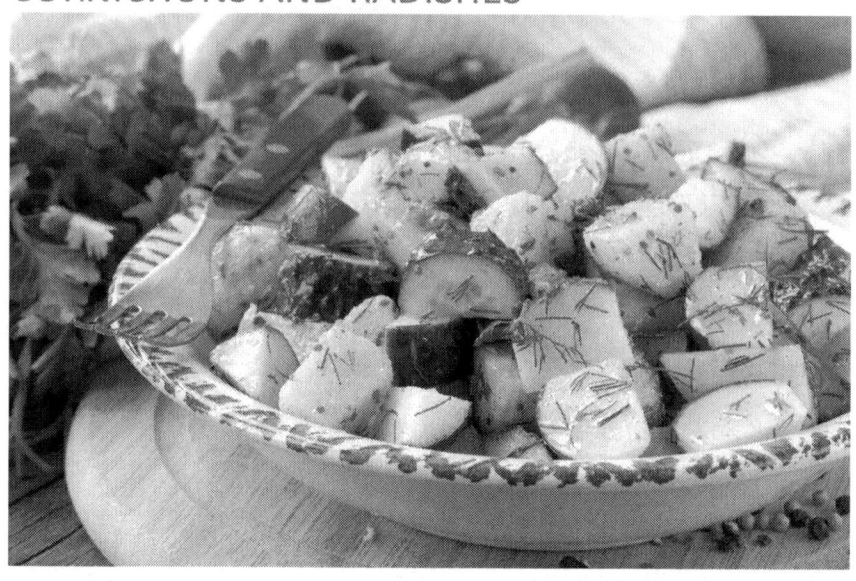

Nutritional Information per 1 Serving:
Energy (calories): 190 kcal
Protein: 2.97 g
Fat: 9.25 g
Carbohydrates: 25.08 g
Gluten-free
Vegan

Ingredients (8 servings):

- 2 lbs. of new potatoes
- 7 oz. of cornichons
- one bunch radishes
- ⅓ cup of chives
- one red onion

Vinaigrette:

- ⅓ cup of neutral oil
- 1 tsp of mustard
- 2 tsp of Dijon mustard
- ⅓ cup of apple cider vinegar
- Salt
- pepper

Directions:

1. Cut the potatoes into thin slices or cut into cubes.
2. Cook potatoes in slightly salted water about 15 minutes.
3. Drain, leave to cool down.
4. Combine all salad ingredients.
5. Put all vinaigrette ingredients in a jar and shake well.
6. Drizzle over the salad then serve.

9. DIETARY LETTUCE SALAD WITH APPLE DRESSING

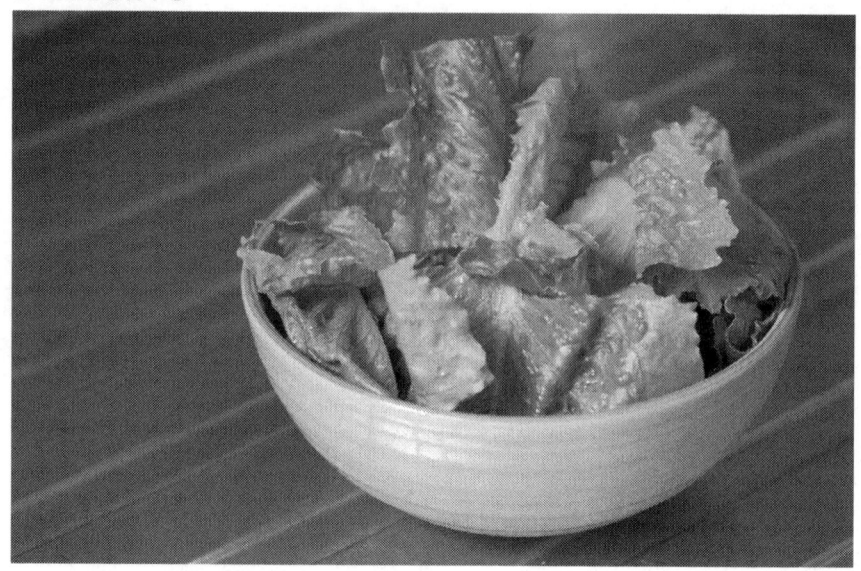

Nutritional Information per 1 Serving:
Energy (calories): 187 kcal
Protein: 1.72 g
Fat: 14.02 g
Carbohydrates: 15.28 g
Gluten-free
Vegan

Ingredients (1 serving):
- Classic apple cider vinegar dressing [Made from the Book]
- 2 cup Pre-made romaine lettuce
- 2 tsp. Apple Cider Vinegar
- 1 Tbs olive oil

Directions:

1. Take 2 Cups of lettuce and mix the apple cider vinegar in with your hands
2. Then drizzle the Apple Cider Vinegar Dressing and olive oil on top

10. FRESH COLLARD GREEN SALAD

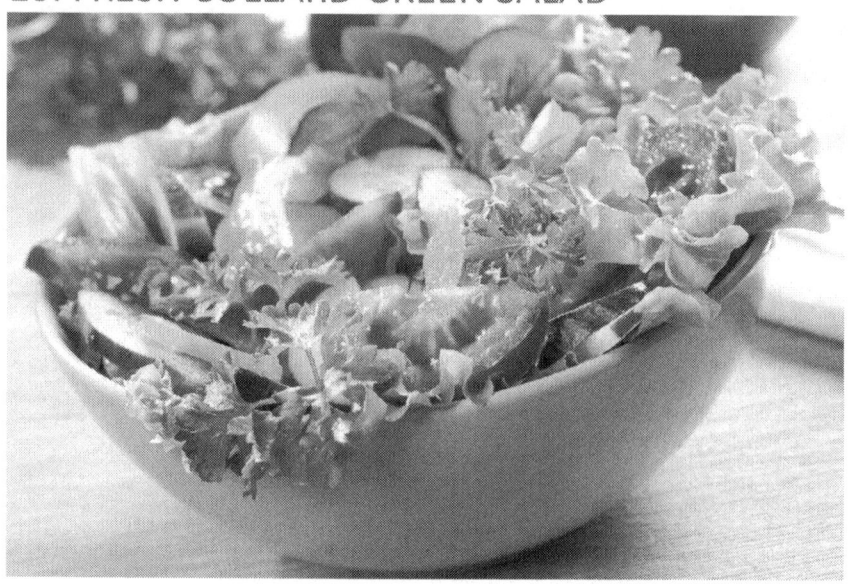

Nutritional Information per 1 Serving:
  Energy (calories): 209 kcal
  Protein: 8.62 g
  Fat: 9.35 g
  Carbohydrates: 28.5 g
  Gluten-free
  Vegan

Ingredients (2 servings):

- 1 lb. of collard greens
- 2 diced tomatoes
- 1 sliced cucumber
- ½ Chopped bell pepper
- 3 Tbsp. of olive oil
- ½ cup of apple cider vinegar
- 2 tsp. of soy sauce (may contain a gluten!)
- 1 tsp. of honey
- salt

- pepper

Directions:

1. Mix in olive oil with collard greens for 5 minutes.
2. Add in peppers.
3. Combine soy sauce, honey, and vinegar; whisk. Drizzle on the peppers and greens; toss.
4. Leave in the fridge for 2 hours.
5. Add tomatoes, cucumber and bell pepper before serving.
6. Flavor using pepper and salt.

11. BRIGHT DETOX SALAD

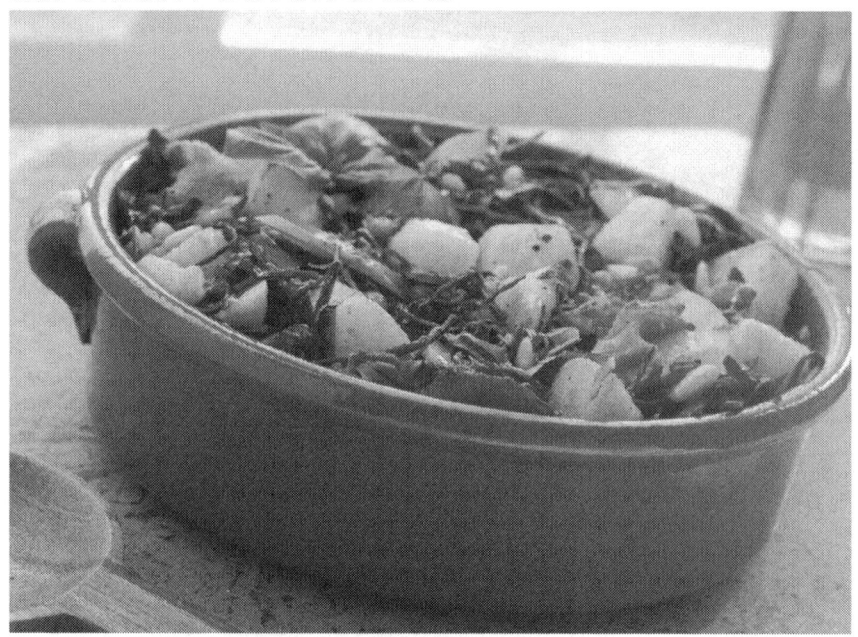

Nutritional Information per 1 Serving:
Energy (calories): 217 kcal
Protein: 6.76 g
Fat: 11.12 g
Carbohydrates: 27.08 g
Gluten-free
Vegan

Ingredients (4 servings):

- 2 sweet potatoes (8 oz.)
- 6 cups of kale
- 2 cups of red cabbage
- one squash (10-12 oz.)
- ⅓ cup of tahini
- ⅓ cup of apple cider vinegar
- ⅓ cup of lemon juice
- 1 tsp. of honey

- 1 tsp. of ginger
- one clove garlic
- 2 tsp. of cilantro
- salt

Directions:

1. Bake the sweet potatoes and the squash. Dice then leave in the fridge to cool.
2. Boil water. Cook the kale for a minute then drain.
3. Leave kale in the fridge till cold.
4. Mix vegetables, stirring in sweet potatoes without mashing.
5. Combine the rest of the ingredients with by a whisk.
6. Drizzle over vegetables; toss well.

12. TASTY WARM POTATO SALAD

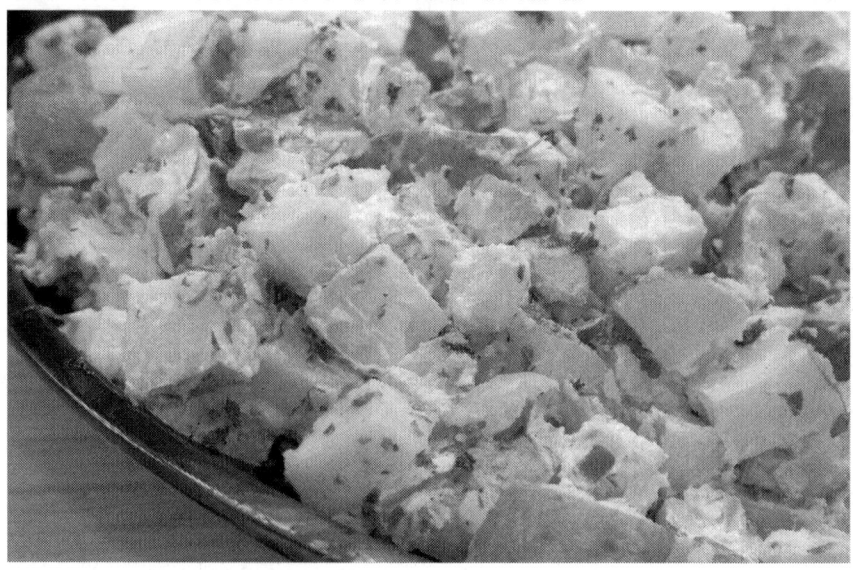

Nutritional Information per 1 Serving:
Energy (calories): 184 kcal
Protein: 3.44 g
Fat: 6.98 g
Carbohydrates: 28.22 g
Gluten-free
Vegan

Ingredients (4 servings):

- 2 ½lbs. of potato (Yukon gold)
- 1 ½Tsp of salt
- one shallot (4 oz.)
- 2 tsp. of spicy brown mustard
- 1 Tbsp. of apple cider vinegar
- 1/4 cup of olive oil
- one tsp of black pepper
- one red pepper
- 2Tbsp. of flat leaf parsley

Directions:

1. Place potatoes in a saucepan and add cold water.
2. Let boil after adding a teaspoon salt. When cooking, simmer over low heat for 10 minutes.
3. Drain and leave to cool down.
4. Combine brown mustard, shallots, apple cider vinegar, half-teaspoon salt then ground black pepper; whisk.
5. While whisking, add in olive oil and emulsify.
6. Mix in the potatoes with the parsley and red peppers.
7. Toss well.

13. FRESH BROCCOLI SALAD FOR LUNCH

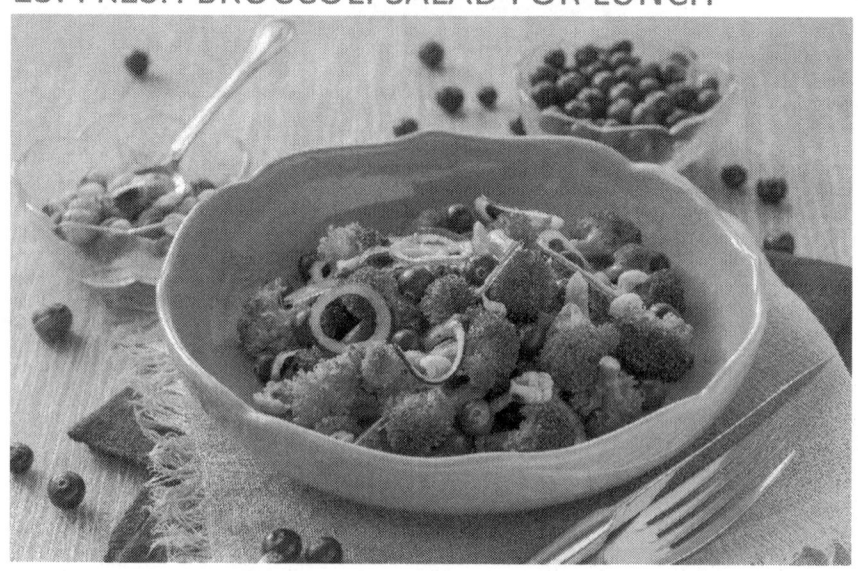

Nutritional Information per 1 Serving:
  Energy (calories): 182 kcal
  Protein: 8.07 g
  Fat: 4.98 g
  Carbohydrates: 31.63 g
  Gluten-free
  Vegan

Ingredients (2 servings):

- 3 Tbs. Apple Cider Vinegar
- ½ Tbs. Olive Oil
- 1 Tbs. Dijon Mustard
- 1 ¼ Tbs. Sugar
- 1/8 tsp. Salt
- ¼ tsp. Black Pepper
- 1 ½ cup Chopped Apples
- ½ cranberries
- ½ cup Onions
- 1 lbs Broccoli

Directions:

1. Mix together all the ingredients.
2. This is a filling salad.
3. If you wish to make it richer, add some dices of meat to it.

MAIN DISHES AND SIDE DISHES
14. DELICATE ALMOND SNACK

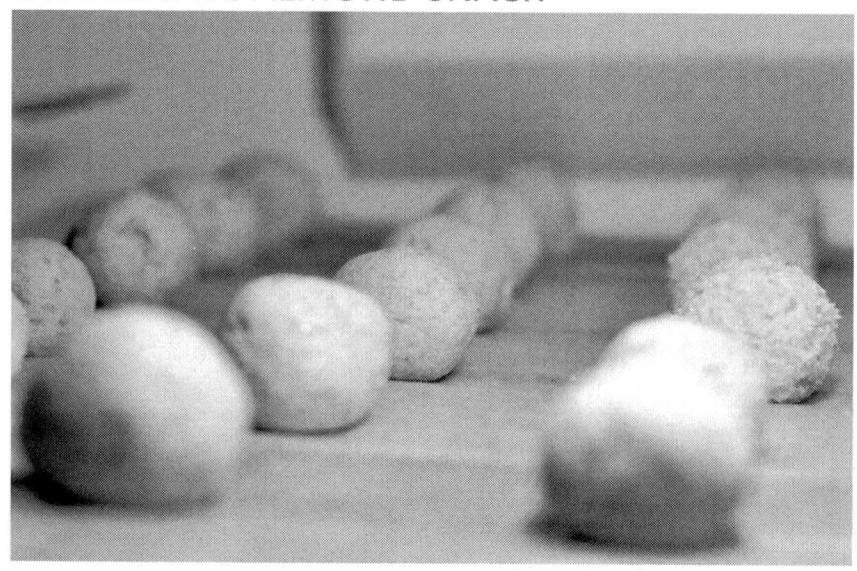

Nutritional Information per 1 Serving:
   Energy (calories): 148 kcal
   Protein: 14.85 g
   Fat: 1.6 g
   Carbohydrates: 19.91 g
   Gluten-free
   Vegan

Ingredients (4 Servings):

- 4 cup Almonds. raw, sprout overnight in enough water to cover
- 3 large Roma tomatoes
- Three ribs celery (6 oz.)
- 2 Tbsp. Apple Cider Vinegar
- 3/4 cup nutritional yeast flakes (do not use powder)
- 1/2 tbsp. cayenne pepper
- 1/2 tbsp. turmeric

- 1/4 cup Aminos (optional)

Directions:

1. Drain and rinse the almonds that have been soaking overnight.
2. Lightly chop almonds first in a food processor.
3. Place all other ingredients into the food processor and process until mixture has thick, pate consistency.
4. Pour mixture into a glass or porcelain pate pan or bread pan.
5. Cover with plastic down to the plate and refrigerate overnight to help it set.
6. The consistency of your pate will depend on how long you processed the ingredients and how much liquid was in the vegetables.
7. Scoop out small balls of paste and serve with sliced vegetables.
8. It is a great snack or addition to your meal on the two-day program

15. LAUNCH BURGERS WITH BACON AND PEACH

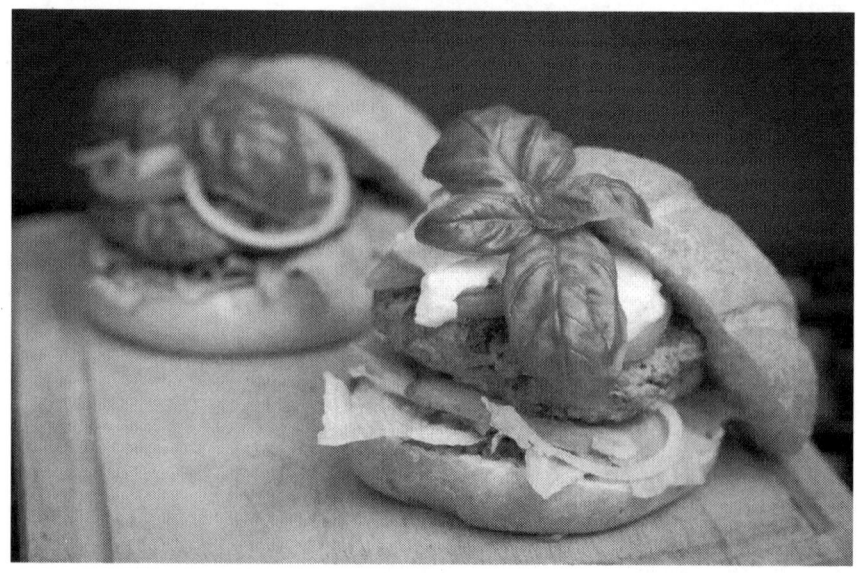

Nutritional Information per 1 Serving:
 Energy (calories): 477 kcal
 Protein: 34.96 g
 Fat: 16.97 g
 Carbohydrates: 46.8 g

Ingredients (4 Servings):

- 1 lb. Ground beef
- 1/2 bell pepper
- 1/2 tsp of chili powder
- 1 oz of goat cheese
- salt
- pepper Peach chutney
- 2 thick bacon slices
- 1/2 onion
- 1 garlic clove
- 1/2 cup of peach preserves

- 1 Tbsp of apple cider vinegar
- 1/2 tsp of chili powder
- 1/4 tsp of ginger

Serving:

- hamburger buns
- 1 peach
- basil leaves

Directions:

1. Preheat your grill to 350 to 400 °F. mix pepper, chili powder and beef.
2. Split meat mix into four and mold around rounds of goat cheese to create four patties.
3. Flavor with pepper and salt.
4. Cook bacon until crisp and then drain using paper towels.
5. Set aside tablespoon bacon drippings to sauté onion and garlic in.
6. Add apple cider vinegar, seasonings, and preserves. Set aside.
7. Grill patties for 4-5 minutes per side.
8. Serve patties using toasted buns alongside bacon, onion mixture, peach slices, tomatoes, basil leaves.

16. FAVORITE BBQ CHICKEN WITH A PEACHES

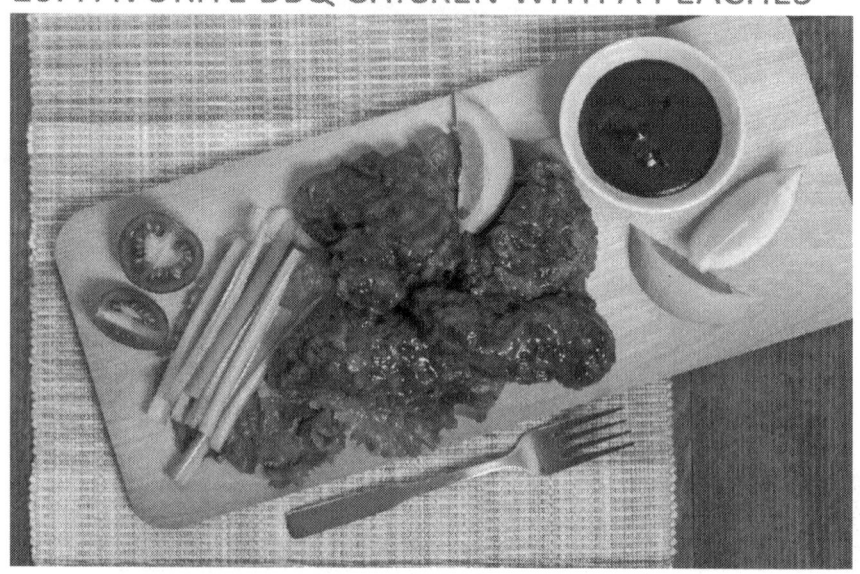

Nutritional Information per 1 Serving:
Energy (calories): 351 kcal
Protein: 24.51 g
Fat: 24.24 g
Carbohydrates: 8.12 g
Gluten-free

Ingredients (6 Servings):
- 2 lbs. of chicken thighs
- ½ cup of BBQ sauce (may contain a gluten!)
- one garlic clove
- 2 Tbsp. of apple cider vinegar
- ½ tsp of paprika
- ½ tsp of chili powder
- two peaches
- rice or another garnish
- cilantro

Directions:

1. Cook chicken using a slow cooker.
2. Mix vinegar, spices, BBQ sauce, and garlic; stir to combine.
3. Mash peaches.
4. Stir in BBQ sauce and peaches onto the slow cooker.
5. Keep cooking on high for at least 3 hours.
6. When done, shred chicken.
7. Put back chicken into the crock pot and mix with left over juice.
8. Top garnish with the chicken and a sprinkling of cilantro.

17. FANTASTIC HEALTHY LUNCH WITH SWEET FIGS

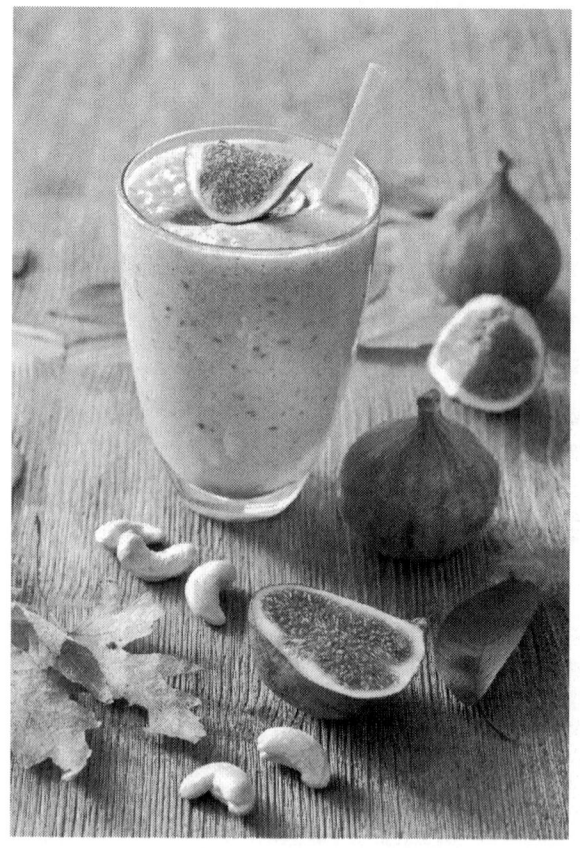

Nutritional Information per 1 Serving:
Energy (calories): 183 kcal
Protein: 3.79 g
Fat: 3.34 g
Carbohydrates: 37.58 g
Gluten-free
Vegan

Ingredients (8 Servings):

- 1 cup of raw buckwheat groats
- 3 cups of water
- 1 ½ Tbsp of apple cider vinegar

- ½ cup of almond milk
- ¼ cup of pure maple syrup
- 1 Tbsp of almond butter
- 1 Tbsp of chia seeds
- ½ Tbsp of coconut oil
- 1 tsp of vanilla extract
- ½ tsp of cinnamon
- Cardamom

Rhubarb compote:

- 1½ cups of rhubarb
- 1 Tbsp of pure maple syrup
- 1 Tbsp of water
- ¼ tsp of cardamom

Garnishe green figs and pepitas

Directions:

1. Soak buckwheat groats in 2 to 3 cups water with apple cider vinegar. Leave overnight in the fridge or for 8 hours.
2. After soaking, strain and rinse well.
3. Using a blender, pulse groats with chia seeds, coconut oil, almond milk, cinnamon, cardamom, almond butter, maple syrup, and vanilla extract,
4. Rhubarb Compote Prep: Cook together maple syrup, sliced rhubarb, water, and cardamom over medium to high heat for 10 to 12 minutes.

Options: The compote can be layered the on the porridge or blend in with buckwheat.

5. After pouring some into the glass, top using pepitas and figs.
6. Leave in the fridge if not serving immediately.

18. TENDER EASY DUCK CARNITAS

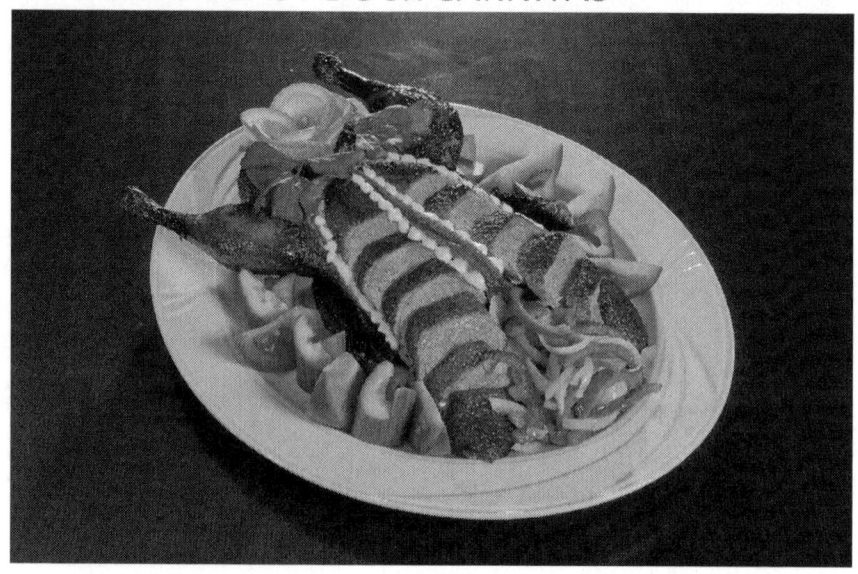

Nutritional Information per 1 Serving:
  Energy (calories): 226 kcal
  Protein: 25.3 g
  Fat: 10.71 g
  Carbohydrates: 6.47 g
  Gluten-free

Ingredients (4 Servings):

- 4 duck legs
- 1 tsp of salt
- 1 tsp of smoked paprika
- 1 tsp of Aleppo pepper
- 1/2 tsp of cumin seed
- 1/2 tsp of Mexican oregano
- 1 navel orange
- 1 cup of water
- 1 tbsp of apple cider vinegar

Directions:

1. Heat oven: 350°F.
2. Using an oven-safe pot, Arrange duck legs with the skins-side-up.
3. Season using all the spices, apple cider vinegar and squeeze orange juice over it.
4. Add water and cover.
5. Let the duck cook (braise) 1 ½ hours.
6. After, remove cover and roast for 1 hour.
7. Shred meat minus the bones and skin when done.
8. Serve with cilantro, wedges and pickled onions.

19. SWEET BROCCOLI WITH PINE NUTS

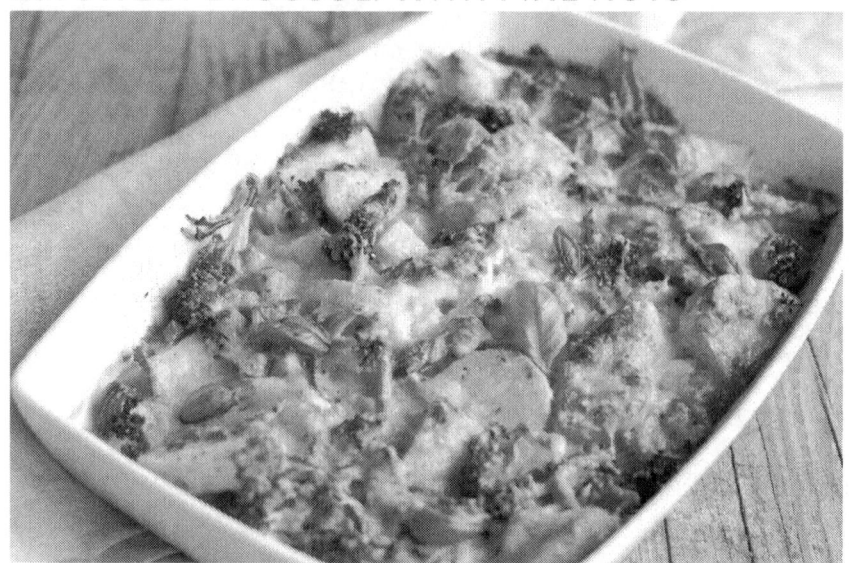

Nutritional Information per 1 Serving:
  Energy (calories): 183 kcal
  Protein: 5.06 g
  Fat: 14.08 g
  Carbohydrates: 11.83 g
  Gluten-free

Ingredients (8 Servings):
- 6 Cups broccoli florets, small
- 2 ½ Cups cauliflower florets, small
- 2 potatoes, chopped
- 1 Tbs canola oil
- 1 tsp salt (to taste)
- 1 tsp ground ginger
- 1 tsp ground cumin
- 1 tsp ground coriander
- 1 tsp freshly ground nutmeg
- 1 tsp crushed red pepper flakes (to taste)
- 2 Cup sour cream
- 2 Tbs. Apple Cider Vinegar

- 1 Tbs mild honey (to taste)
- 1 Cup thinly sliced green onions
- 1 Cup toasted pine nuts

Directions:
1. Preheat oven to 350°F
2. Mix together all the ingredients and put in a baking dish
3. Then bake about 30 minutes
4. Remove from the oven and serve

20. CREAMY VEGAN MUSHROOM STROGANOFF

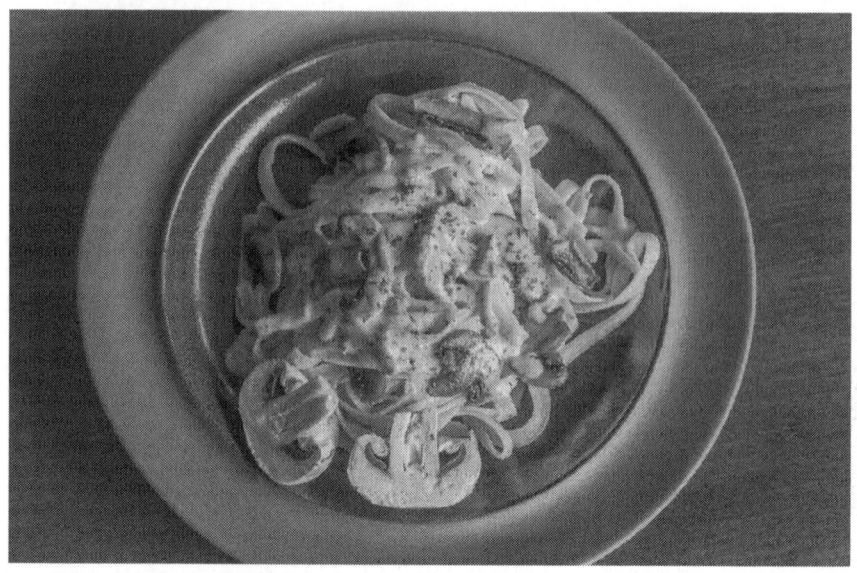

Nutritional Information per 1 Serving:
Energy (calories): 315 kcal
Protein: 6.52 g
Fat: 17.25 g
Carbohydrates: 37.76 g
Gluten-free
Vegan

Ingredients (8 Servings):

- 1 package of Gluten-free Fettuccini
- 2 lbs. Portobello mushrooms
- ½ cup of veggie broth
- ½ cup of almond milk
- 2 Tbsp. of apple cider vinegar
- 1 Tbsp. of nutritional yeast
- 1 Tbsp. of miso paste
- 2 tsp of soy sauce (may contain a gluten!)

- ½ tsp of nutmeg
- ½ tsp of cayenne pepper
- ¼ tsp of liquid smoke
- Salt
- pepper
- basil

Directions:

1. Slice mushrooms thinly.
2. Combine the liquid smoke, a teaspoon veggie broth, and soy sauce; whisk. Stir in mushrooms and toss.
3. Let mushrooms marinate for 30 minutes.
4. Add the rest of ingredients minus the pasta with the mushrooms on a saucepan and let boil about 10-15 minutes.
5. Simmer the sauce over low heat.
6. Cook fettuccini.
7. Drain fettuccini and pour sauce, tossing well to combine.
8. Garnish with torn basil leaves.

21. PICKLED "FRIED" GREEN TOMATOES WITH CREAMY-HERB SAUCE

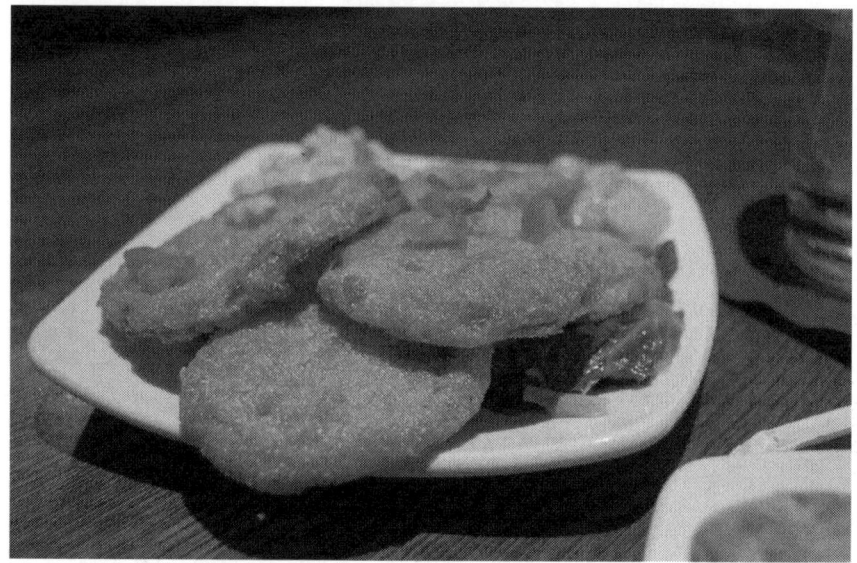

Nutritional Information per 1 Serving:
Energy (calories): 244 kcal
Protein: 9.78 g
Fat: 6.86 g
Carbohydrates: 38.32 g

Ingredients (8 servings):

- 1 cup of water
- 1 cup of apple cider vinegar
- 1 Tbs. of sugar
- ½ Tbs. of salt
- 16 green Tomatoes
- 5 Tbs. of buttermilk
- 1 Tbs. of olive oil mayonnaise
- 1 Tbs. of dill
- 2 Tbs. of apple cider vinegar
- 1 clove garlic
- ½ tsp of black pepper

- 1¼ cup of panko (breadcrumbs)
- ⅓ cup of masa haring
- ¼ tsp of salt
- 1 egg
- 1 egg white
- ¼ cup of flour
- tbsp of EV olive oil
- 6 oz. Mozzarella cheese for serving or goat cheese

Directions:
1. Let boil all picking ingredients. Add in the tomatoes and keep cooking for 2 minutes. When done, leave for 15 min, drain and pat dry.
2. Mix next 4 of ingredients up to garlic with five tablespoons buttermilk; whisk. Add ¼-teaspoon pepper.
3. Toast panko for 2 minutes. Remove from fire and add ¼-teaspoon salt, masa haring, and ¼-teaspoon pepper. Mix egg, egg white, two tablespoons buttermilk; stir. Put flour in a separate dish.
4. Coat tomato slices using flour first, dip in the egg mixture and lastly coat with the panko.
5. Cook half of the tomatoes over medium to high heat until browned. Do the same with the rest of the vegetables and serve with the sauce and Mozzarella cheese.

SOUPS
22. RED VEGETABLE SOUP

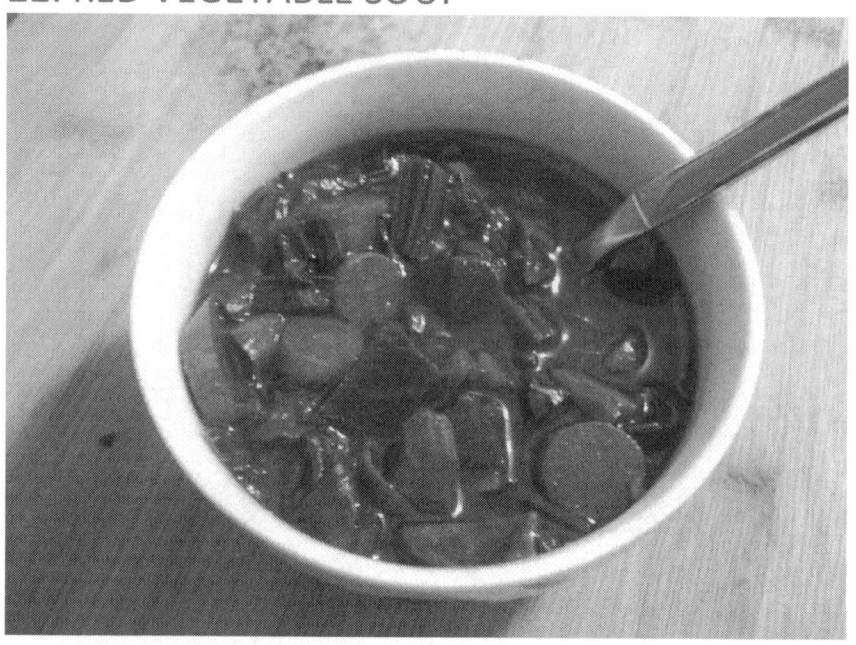

Nutritional Information per 1 Serving:
Energy (calories): 69 kcal
Protein: 1.45 g
Fat: 1.24 g
Carbohydrates: 14.23 g
Gluten-free
Vegan

Ingredients (6 servings):

- 1 Sweet Potato
- 1 Carrot
- ½ Beet
- ½ diced Onion
- 1 Parsnip
- 6 cups of Water
- ¼ cup of Apple Cider Vinegar

- 1 Tbs Olive Oil to sauté
- A pinch of Salt

Directions:

1. After washing all the vegetable thoroughly cut them into large chunks. Now put the onions in a pot and sauté it in olive oil until fragrant.
2. Now slip in the carrots, beets, sweet potato and parsnip and mix it well. Then start adding water to the mixture to fully submerge the vegetables.
3. Leave it to boil and let the mixture simmer. Taste it once to see if the soup has the desired taste or not.
4. Once the vegetables are tender and the taste is accordance with your needs, remove the soup from heat and add the ACV and a pinch of salt.

23. NON-FAT DELICIOUS SOUP

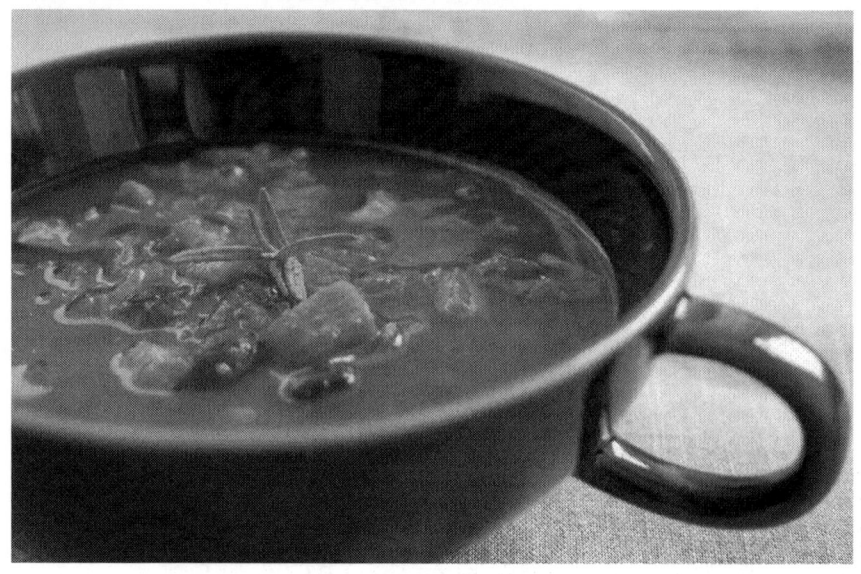

Nutritional Information per 1 Serving:
Energy (calories): 145 kcal
Protein: 5.83 g
Fat: 4.75 g
Carbohydrates: 22.38 g
Gluten-free
Vegan

Ingredients (8 servings):
- 4 Cups nonfat vegetable broth or 4 Cups vegetarian chicken broth
- 2 Cups diced onions
- 2 Cups diced celery
- 2 Cups peeled and diced carrots
- 1 Cup green beans (or asparagus, Brussel sprouts, eggplant, cauliflower)
- 1 ½ Cups finely chopped green cabbage (or try spinach, swiss chard, or other greens)

- 1 Cup diced red bell peppers (may sub green peppers okra)
- 1 summer squash
- 4 garlic cloves, minced
- 3 Cups diced tomatoes with juice (28 oz. can)
- 2 Tbs. soy sauce (may contain a gluten!)
- 1 Tbsp. Apple Cider Vinegar 3 Tbs. paprika
- 1 tsp dried basil
- 1 tsp dried oregano
- 1 tsp dried dill
- 1/2 tsp dried thyme
- 1/2 tsp ground black pepper salt

Directions:

1. Pour broth into a pot and bring to a boil.
2. Add in onions, basil, paprika, oregano and dill.
3. Stir for 2-3 minutes.
4. Then add in thyme, pepper, and Apple Cider Vinegar.
5. Stir for 1 minute.
6. Add the rest of the ingredients until the carrots are soft.
7. This will leave the cabbage slightly crunchy and still give that refreshing taste to cool down the paprika.

24. DELIGHT BROWN RICE SOUP WITH LENTIL

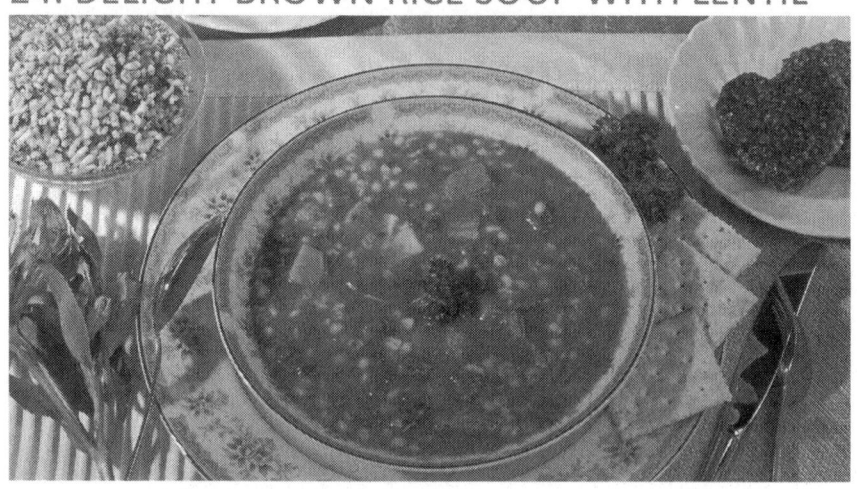

Nutritional Information per 1 Serving:
Energy (calories): 311 kcal
Protein: 20.75 g
Fat: 16.33 g
Carbohydrates: 26.76 g
Gluten-free

Ingredients (8 servings):
- 5 Cups chicken broth
- 3 Cups lentils, picked over and rinsed
- 1 Cup cooked brown rice
- 1 (2 lb.) can of tomatoes, drained, reserving juice, and chopped
- 3 carrots, halved lengthwise and cut crosswise into ¼ inch pieces
- 1 onions, chopped
- 1 stalk celery, chopped
- 3 1/2 cloves garlic, minced
- 1/2 tsp crumbled dried basil
- 1/2 Tps crumbled oregano
- 1/4 Tps crumbled dried thyme

- 1 bay leaf
- 1/2 Cup minced fresh parsley
- 3 Tbs. Apple Cider Vinegar
- 1 1/2 lb smoked sausage

Directions:
1. Turn the stove on medium-high.
2. Combine broth, 3 ½ Cups water, lentils, tomatoes, carrots, onion, celery, herbs and sausage and bring to boil.
3. Simmer for about 30 minutes and then add in brown rice.
4. Simmer until lentils are tender for another 30 minutes.
5. Add the Apple Cider Vinegar.

HEALTHY TASTY SMOOTHIES
25. GREEN APPLE CIDER VINEGAR SMOOTHIE

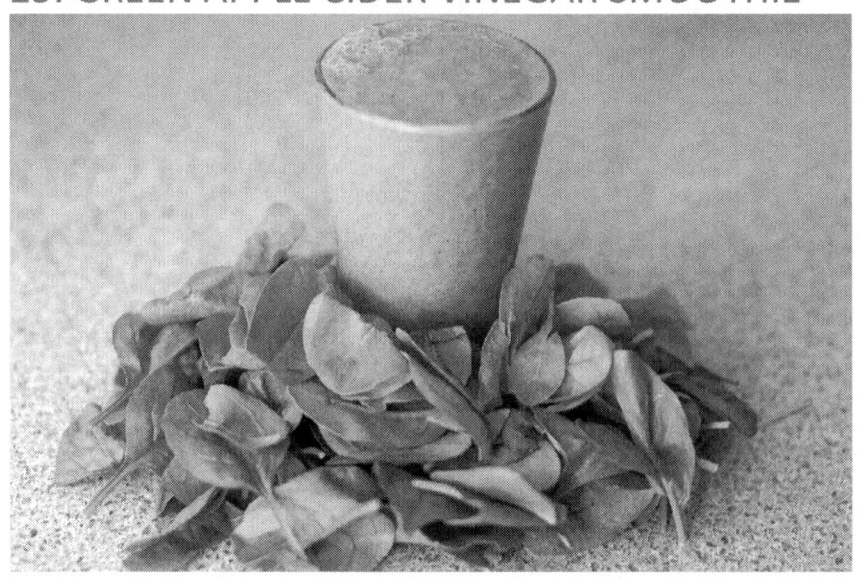

Nutritional Information per 1 Serving:
 Energy (calories): 205 kcal
 Protein: 9.24 g
 Fat: 0.83 g
 Carbohydrates: 44.05 g
 Gluten-free

Ingredients (4 servings):
- 4 handfuls of Baby Spinach
- 2 Bananas (sliced)
- 2 Apples (diced)
- 2 cups of Yogurt
- 10 Strawberries
- 1 Orange
- 2 Tbs. Apple Cider Vinegar

Directions:
1. Give a good Blend to these ingredients.
2. In the end, you will have a delicious green smoothie.

26. SUNNY MANGO SMOOTHIE WITH APPLE CIDER VINEGAR

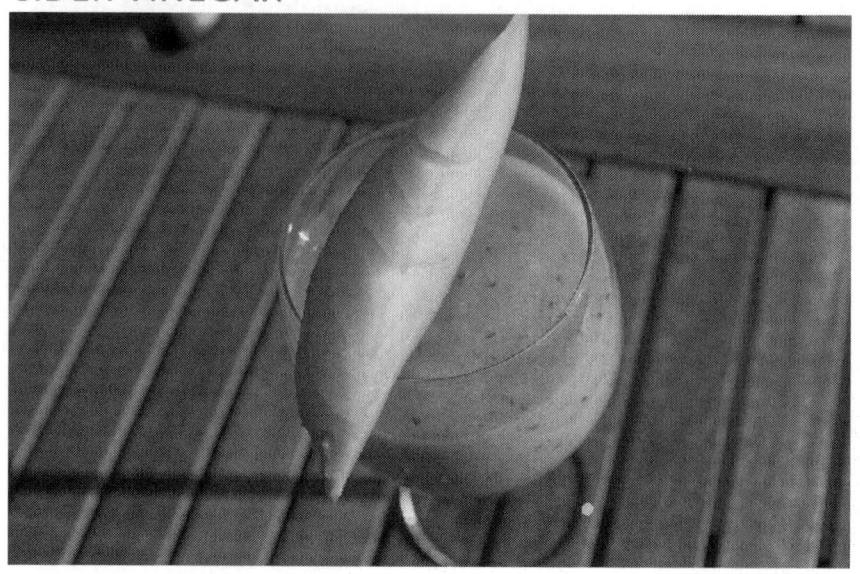

Nutritional Information per 1 Serving:
Energy (calories): 175 kcal
Protein: 2.27 g
Fat: 2.69 g
Carbohydrates: 37.69 g
Gluten-free
Vegan

Ingredients (2 servings):
- 1 cup Mangoes (sliced)
- 1 Banana (sliced)
- ½ cup of Orange Juice
- ½ tsp. Vanilla Extract
- ¼ cup Ice Cubes
- 1 Tbs. of Apple Cider Vinegar
- A pinch of ground Cinnamon

Directions:
1. Blend all the ingredients together until smooth.
2. Prepare this delicious smoothie in under 10 minutes.

27. APPLE CIDER VINEGAR DETOX SMOOTHIE

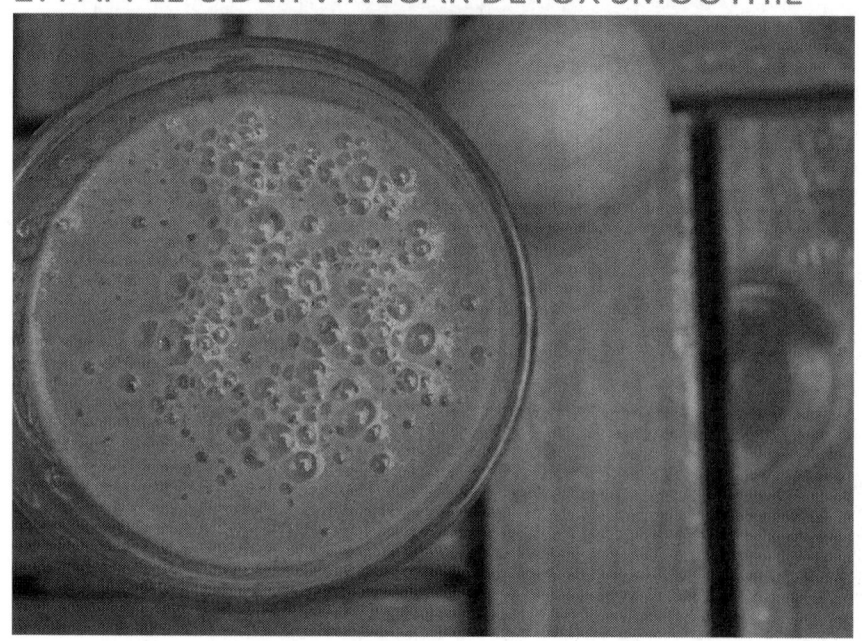

Nutritional Information per 1 Serving:
 Energy (calories): 163 kcal
 Protein: 1.96 g
 Fat: 0.81 g
 Carbohydrates: 41.83 g
 Gluten-free
 Vegan

Ingredients (2 servings):

- 2 Tbs. of Ginger juice
- 3 Green Apples (chopped)
- 1 Tbs. Lime Juice
- 1 Tbs. of Apple Cider Vinegar
- Handful of Arugula
- 5 Ice Cubes
- Stevia to taste

Directions:
1. Throw all the ingredients in a blender and mix them well.
2. Blend until smooth.
3. Serve it fresh.

28. MILKY BANANA SMOOTHIE WITH KALE

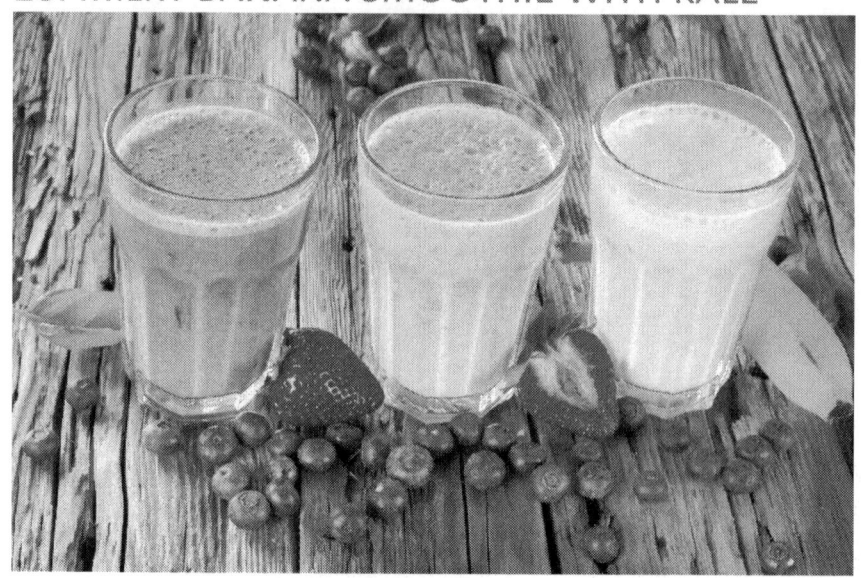

Nutritional Information per 1 Serving:
 Energy (calories): 195 kcal
 Protein: 3.62 g
 Fat: 2.26 g
 Carbohydrates: 44.7 g
 Gluten-free
 Vegan

Ingredients (2 servings):

- 1 Banana (sliced)
- 1 cup Almond Milk
- ¼ tsp. of Cinnamon
- 15 Blueberries or 10 Strawberries
- ½ Tbs. of Ginger (juice)
- 1 Tbs. of Honey
- 1 small bunch of Kale
- 1 Tbs. of Apple Cider Vinegar

Directions:
1. Blend all the ingredients together until smooth.
2. This drink can also be considered as a detoxifying smoothie.

29. DELICIOUS ENERGY FRUIT SMOOTHIE

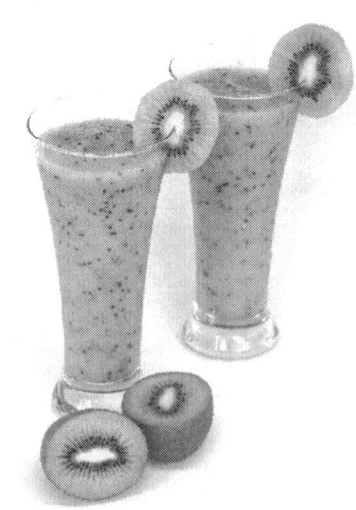

Nutritional Information per 1 Serving:
  Energy (calories): 168 kcal
  Protein: 1.61 g
  Fat: 0.53 g
  Carbohydrates: 43.36 g
  Gluten-free
  Vegan

Ingredients (2 servings):

- 1 Banana
- 1 Kiwi, skinned
- ½ package of pre-cut apple (2 apples)
- 2 tsp. Apple Cider Vinegar
- 1 tsp sugar or Stevia to taste

Directions:
1. Put into a blender and blend until smooth.

CONCLUSION

Thank you for purchasing this book. I hope you will apply the acquired knowledge productively. I personally feel the struggle of being Apple cider vinegar-obsessed, but often disappointed by boring, same or downright dry and tasteless apple cider recipes. If you're in the same boat, look no further! It's time to take control and start making our own sweet and delicious dishes at home using the apple cider vinegar. With recipes for all occasions or seasons, ranging from the perfect-for-winter to the light and summer. Join me on the transformation journey to discover your inner cooking and to create some downright delicious apple cider vinegar recipes. Let's get cooking!

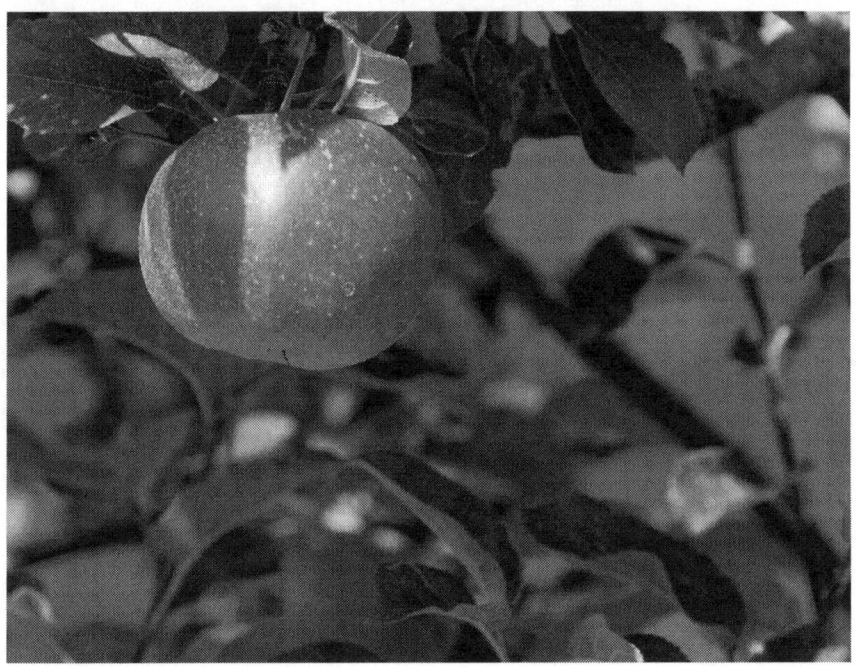

Made in the USA
Lexington, KY
24 June 2019